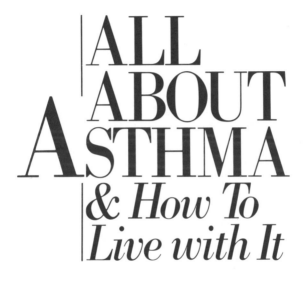

ALL
ABOUT
ASTHMA
& *How To*
Live with It

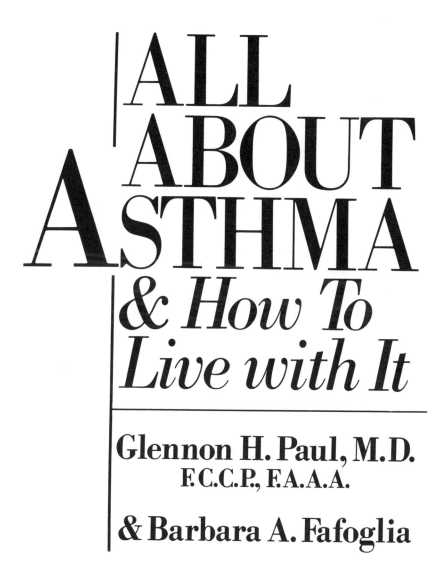

ALL ABOUT ASTHMA

& *How To Live with It*

Glennon H. Paul, M.D.
F.C.C.P., F.A.A.A.

& Barbara A. Fafoglia

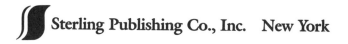 Sterling Publishing Co., Inc.   New York

Edited by Laurel Ornitz

Library of Congress Cataloging-in-Publication Data

Paul, Glennon H.
All about asthma & how to live with it : the complete guide to
understanding and controlling asthma / Glennon H. Paul, Barbara A.
Fafoglia.
p. cm.
Includes index.
ISBN 0-8069-6808-7. ISBN 0-8069-6809-5 (pbk.)
1. Asthma—Popular works. I. Fafoglia, Barbara A. II. Title.
III. Title: All about asthma and how to live with it.
RC591.P38 1988
616.2'38—dc 19   88-2980
                                                                       CIP

5   7   9   10   8   6

Copyright © 1988 by Glennon H. Paul, M.D. & Barbara A. Fafoglia
Published by Sterling Publishing Co., Inc.
387 Park Avenue South, New York, N.Y. 10016
Distributed in Canada by Sterling Publishing
% Canadian Manda Group, P.O. Box 920, Station U
Toronto, Ontario, Canada M8Z 5P9
Distributed in Great Britain and Europe by Cassell PLC
Artillery House, Artillery Row, London SW1P 1RT, England
Distributed in Australia by Capricorn Ltd.
P.O. Box 665, Lane Cove, NSW 2066
Manufactured in the United States of America
All rights reserved
Sterling ISBN 0-8069-6808-7   Trade
          0-8069-6809-5   Paper

Contents

ACKNOWLEDGMENTS   10

DEDICATION   11

NOTE TO THE READERS   12

Understanding Asthma—Causes, Types, and Triggers

1   An Introduction to Asthma—Basic Facts and Statistics   14

2   Understanding Extrinsic (Allergic) Asthma   19
  - *Allergy and Our Immune System*
  - *Common Allergic Triggers: Pollens, Moulds, House Dust, Animal Danders, Insects, Foods, Sulfites, and Drugs*

3   Understanding Intrinsic (Nonallergic) Asthma   35
  - *Similarities and Differences Between Intrinsic and Extrinsic Asthma*
  - *Common Nonallergic Triggers: Irritating Substances, Infections, Stress, Exercise, and Environmental Factors*

4   Understanding Asthma in
    Children   43

- *Facts about Childhood Asthma*
- *Similarities and Differences Between Adult and Childhood Asthma*
- *How To Determine Whether Your Child Is a Mild, Moderate, or Severe Asthmatic*
- *Common Triggers of Asthma in Children*
- *Growth and Development in Children with Asthma*
- *How To Differentiate Asthma from Other Common Respiratory Conditions of Childhood*
- *Physical and Emotional Aspects of Childhood Asthma*
- *Educational Resources Available for Children with Asthma*

Diagnosing Asthma in Adults and Children

5   A Visit to the Allergist—Diagnosing
    Asthma in Children and Adults   58

- *How To Prepare for the Visit*
- *How Asthma Is Diagnosed—Skin Tests, Pulmonary Function Tests, and Laboratory Tests*

6   Asthma, Bronchitis, and Emphysema—
    How To Tell the Difference   68

Caring for Asthma (in General and at Special Times)

7   Medications and Asthma   76

- *Basic Asthma Drugs*
- *When and How To Take Them*
- *How They Work*
- *How They Interact with Food and Drink and Other Drugs*

8   Treating and Controlling Your Asthma   102

- *Treatment Measures*
- *Control with Medicines*
- *Environmental Control*
- *Allergy Shots*
- *Self-Help Techniques*

9   Surgery, Anesthesia, and Asthma   119

- *What To Do Before Surgery To Lessen Problems*
- *How Asthma Medications Affect Anesthesia*
- *How Anesthesia and Surgery Affect Asthma*
- *Safe Anesthetics for Asthma*
- *Preventing Postoperative Complications*
- *Dental Surgery and Asthma*

10   Pregnancy and Asthma   125

- *How They Can Peacefully Coexist*

- *Effects of Asthma on Pregnancy*
- *Effects of Drugs on the Fetus*
- *Breast Feeding and Asthma Drugs*
- *Possible Prevention of Allergy Through Breast Feeding*

11 Asthma Out of Control 133
- *How It's Managed in the Hospital*
- *Complications and Death*

Living with Asthma

12 Asthma at School 146
- *Common Problems at School Faced by Asthmatics—and the Solutions to These Problems*
- *A Team Effort—Tips for Parents, Children, and Teachers*

13 Exercise, Sports, and Asthma 156
- *How To Recognize Exercise-Induced Asthma*
- *How To Treat and Control It*

14 Asthma and the Workplace 162
- *Facts about Occupational Asthma*
- *Causes of Occupational Asthma*
- *Who Can Get It*
- *Prevention Measures*

15 Stress, Hyperventilation, and Asthma 177

- *How to Recognize Stress and Hyperventilation*
- *How Stress, Hyperventilation, and Asthma Are Interrelated*
- *Self-Help Strategies for Stress Management in Controlling Hyperventilation and Asthma*

Appendices

A The Respiratory System and How It Works   190

B Pollens Causing Allergy, and Where They're Found in the United States and Canada   196

C Moulds Triggering Asthma   207

D Food Families   208

E Asthma Breathing Aids, and How To Use Them   211

F Asthma Day or Resident Camps for Children in the United States   213

G Products for Treating Allergy, and Where To Find Them   219

GLOSSARY   223
ABOUT THE AUTHORS   231
INDEX   234

Acknowledgments

We wish to give special thanks to Jim Rostron for creating the illustrations that accompany the text. Also, we wish to extend special thanks to Barb Raye, who diligently worked on word-processing the text. We offer these two people our gratitude for their tenacity and dedication.

Dedication

This book is dedicated to Paul P. Van Arsdel, M.D.; C. Warren Bierman, M.D.; James E. Stroh, Sr., M.D.; James E. Stroh, Jr., M.D.; Rick L. Johnson, M.D.; Stanley J. Zeitz, M.D.; and William E. Pierson, M.D.

Note to the Readers

Knowledge is power, and this book is meant to give you knowledge about asthma to empower you so that you can be an active participant in the management of your asthma. It is not intended to be a substitute for your own doctor's treatment program. Any medication or treatment program discussed in this book should be undertaken only under your doctor's supervision. We hope this book will enable you to become a partner with your doctor so that you can work together in conquering your asthma.

Understanding Asthma

Causes, Types, and Triggers

1

An Introduction to Asthma—Basic Facts and Statistics

1.   About 10 million Americans are known to have asthma: This is about 4 percent of the population.

2.   The number of Americans who have ever had asthma, although they may no longer be symptomatic, is approximately 16 million, or 7 percent of the entire population.

3.   About 5 percent of the asthmatic population experiences severe, recurring attacks.

4.   There are approximately 27 million patient visits to physicians each year for the treatment of asthma.

5.   Every year asthma accounts for an estimated 12 million days spent in bed rest and 24 million days spent in restricted activity.

6.   Asthma is responsible for more than 2 million days of hospitalization each year.

7.   The yearly estimated economic cost of asthma in the United States averages nearly 2.5 billion dollars. This figure includes the cost of hospital admissions, physicians and other health-care providers, drugs and other medications, as well as the indirect costs to society of morbidity and mortality.

8.   Asthma is the most common of all severe lung diseases of childhood.

9.   Asthma is the number one leading cause of time loss from school due to chronic illness, accounting for about 25 percent of such absences.

10.   There are nearly 5,000 documented deaths from asthma per year, and asthma is a contributing cause in an additional 2,000 deaths per year.

11.   Asthma can affect people in any age group and from all walks of life.

12. Asthma is a lung disease that usually can be controlled, and sometimes cured.

What Is Asthma and What Are Its Symptoms?

Asthma is a condition of the bronchial tubes characterized by episodes of constriction and increased mucous production. A person with asthma has bronchial tubes that are supersensitive to various stimuli, or triggers, that can produce asthma symptoms. This means that asthmatics have a special sensitivity that causes their lung tissue to react far more than it should to various stimulating factors, or triggers. For this reason, people with asthma are said to have "twitchy airways."

Asthmatics commonly experience such symptoms as chest tightness, difficulty inhaling and exhaling, wheezing, production of large amounts of mucus in their windpipes, and coughing. Coughing can be frequent or intermittent, and can be loose—reflecting extra mucous secretion in the airways—or dry and deep—reflecting tight bronchospasms. Not all of these symptoms occur in every case of asthma. Sometimes people may have coughing without any other symptoms for months or even years before it's realized that they are asthmatic. Interestingly enough, most asthma symptoms become more severe at night.

Why Are Asthma Symptoms More Severe At Night?

Asthma is worse at night because when we lie down our airways narrow as a result of gravity changes. Also, our lungs do not clear secretions as well at night, which leads to mucous retention, and that can increase the obstruction to airflow. Furthermore, at night our bodies produce smaller amounts of certain chemicals that help to decrease airway spasms and keep airway tubes open. All of these factors add up to a greater chance of symptoms worsening at night.

What Happens During an Asthma Attack?

An asthma attack begins when the smooth muscles in the walls of the bronchial tubes start to tighten and narrow when they are exposed to a trigger. When this bronchospasm occurs, air can't flow into or out of the lungs. To make matters worse, mucus enters the narrowed bronchial tubes and plugs them up, causing a further decrease in airflow. The bronchial tubes seem to close down, and air moving through these narrowed breathing passages can cause wheezing (high-pitched, whistlelike sounds). Wheezing can be loud enough to be heard across a room, or it can be so slight that it takes a stethoscope to hear it. Airflow obstruction leads to air trapping in the lungs. This trapped, stale air builds up in the lungs, increasing respiratory distress by leaving little space for fresh air. With less fresh air available, there is less oxygen available to fuel our bodies.

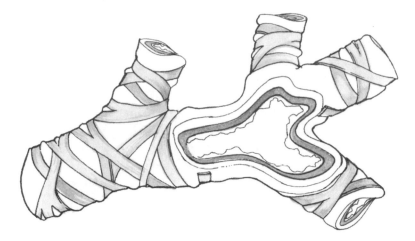

Normal bronchial tube with very little mucus and no narrowing.

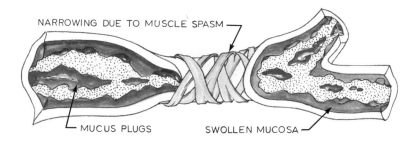

This is what a bronchial tube looks like when an individual has asthma. The bronchial tubes in asthma are narrowed due to muscle spasm and swollen mucous membranes (mucosa), and are often plugged with mucus.

How Severe Can Asthma Become?

Asthma attacks can be so mild they're hardly noticed or so severe that asthmatics can feel like they're suffocating. Although more attacks seem to occur at night, they can virtually happen anytime. Attacks may come on very suddenly, or they may develop slowly over a period of hours or days. Some asthmatics are relatively symptom-free between attacks, whereas others having chronic asthma live with symptoms every day. These symptoms can vary from mild irritation to extreme interference in one's ability to perform life's daily functions. Severe asthmatics often require hospitalization and continuous, aggressive medical and allergic treatment for asthma control. Although the severe asthmatic group is at a greater risk of death from their disease, it is important to realize that most deaths from asthma can be avoided with proper treatment.

What Triggers Asthma?

Among other contributing factors, asthmatics have an imbalance in the part of their autonomic nervous system that controls the reactivity of their windpipes. This imbalance causes their windpipes to become overreactive to many different stimulating factors, or triggers. An asthmatic trigger can be any stimulus that brings about or sets off asthma symptoms. Asthma triggers vary widely among asthmatics. Triggers will be discussed at greater length in Chapters 2 and 3, but for now, we'll categorize the most common triggers into the following groups:

- allergies;
- irritating substances, such as dust, fumes, odors, and vapors;
- environmental factors, including weather changes and air pollution;
- infections (primarily viral infections, such as colds and flu); and
- stress (both positive and negative).

An important step in getting control of your asthma is to discover the factors or combination of factors that trigger your attacks. The more you know about your asthma triggers, the better you will be able to understand asthma and work along with your doctor to prevent or control it.

Does Asthma Run in Families?

If asthma runs in your family, you're likely to have it, too. Consider your chances for having asthma by looking at these statistics:

Family history compared with chances of having asthma

both parents have asthma	*50% chance of asthma in offspring*
one parent has asthma	*25% chance of asthma in offspring*
neither parent has asthma	*less than 10% chance of asthma in offspring*

Allergy also runs in families; consider your chances of having allergy if it runs in your family:

Family history compared with chances of having allergy

both parents have allergy	*65% chance of allergies in offspring*
one parent has allergy	*35% chance of allergies in offspring*
neither parent has allergy	*less than 10% chance of allergies in offspring*

Since allergy is a major asthma trigger, your chances of developing asthma will be even higher if *both* allergy and asthma run in your family.

How Many Kinds of Asthma Exist?

Generally speaking, asthma can be divided into two categories: *extrinsic*, or allergic asthma, which is triggered by allergies; and *intrinsic*, or non-allergic asthma, which is triggered by nonallergic factors. Asthma triggers tend to be extrinsic in younger people and intrinsic in older people. However, for both kinds of asthma, the symptoms are generally the same. The difference lies in the triggers that set off the asthma. To give you a better understanding of the two kinds of asthma and their triggers, we'll discuss each of them separately in the next two chapters.

2
Understanding Extrinsic (Allergic) Asthma

Extrinsic asthma, otherwise known as allergic asthma, is caused or triggered by allergies. People with extrinsic asthma overreact to common allergens in the environment that are typically harmless to the general population. For these people, allergic asthma triggers can present year-round problems or only seasonal bouts of asthma.

What Is an Allergy?

An allergy is an abnormal response in a person who has been exposed to an *allergen*. An allergen is any substance that triggers allergic reactions in people. The tendency to become allergic is inherited.

Many people wonder what causes their allergic symptoms and why they are worse at certain times of the year. Their symptoms occur when an allergen enters the body through breathing, eating, drinking, or by injection or skin contact. When this happens, people who are allergic form antibodies, or protective mechanisms, to the allergens. These antibodies make people become more sensitive to the allergens. There are many kinds of antibodies, but the one most commonly involved in allergic reactions is called the IgE antibody. Once formed, IgE antibodies are found in body tissues, such as the lining of the nose and lungs, or the skin. When an allergen comes in contact with these IgE antibodies, an allergic reaction occurs and causes adverse symptoms in the allergic person. If this reaction takes place in the lungs, asthma hits with all its familiar symptoms—wheezing, coughing, chest tightness, and shortness of breath. These symptoms tend to worsen in spring, late summer, and fall—the common allergy seasons.

To better understand what's going on inside the body with extrinsic asthma, let's take a look at the immune system, which plays a major role in the allergic reaction.

How Is the Immune System Associated with Extrinsic Asthma?

Everyone is born with a natural immune system that protects them from infections and disease. The immune system works constantly to guard our bodies from potentially harmful invaders. When it identifies a foreign substance as harmful, it begins to attack that substance and tries to destroy it by producing fighters, called antibodies. Sometimes it incorrectly identifies a harmless substance as threatening. When this happens, an abnormal immune response (allergic reaction) occurs and results in adverse symptoms that can range from merely annoying to very severe. When these symptoms occur in the lungs, we get asthma.

Here's what happens. An allergen enters the body. It gets into the circulatory system and is carried to various parts of the body. An allergen causes an allergic person to manufacture IgE antibodies (which doesn't happen in a nonallergic person). IgE antibodies attach themselves to *mast* cells, which are abundant in our respiratory systems. When the allergen and antibody combine and react, they cause the mast cell to release strong chemicals (known as mediators), such as histamine, into the surrounding body tissues. These chemicals produce the allergic reaction that, in our lungs, results in tightening of the windpipes and increased mucous production. An asthmatic's airways are very sensitive to the effects of these chemical mediators.

We'll summarize this section by saying that extrinsic asthmatics make an increased amount of IgE antibodies, which results in a greater release of chemical mediators. In addition, their windpipes are more sensitive to chemical mediators. To help you understand what happens inside the body during an allergic asthmatic reaction, we'll sum up the events in five points:

1. An allergen enters the body.

2. In response to this allergen, which would generally be a harmless substance in a nonallergic person, the allergic person makes IgE antibodies.

3. These IgE antibodies attach to mast cells, which are present in the lining of the respiratory system.

4. The allergen meets the IgE antibodies, which are attached to the mast cells, causing the cells to release strong chemical mediators into the surrounding body tissues.

5. The release of these chemical mediators into the allergic asthmatic's lungs causes tightening in the windpipes and extra mucous production, resulting in asthma.

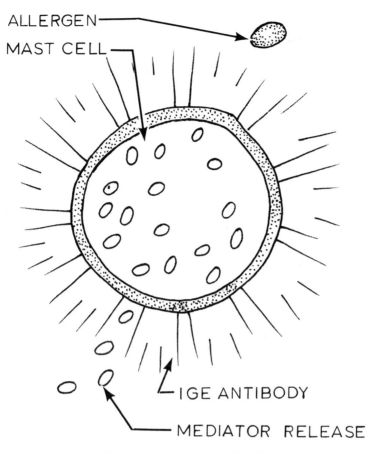

ALLERGEN

MAST CELL

IGE ANTIBODY

MEDIATOR RELEASE

This drawing shows an allergen reacting with an IgE antibody attached to a mast cell, thereby stimulating harmful chemical mediator release, which results in an allergic reaction.

What Are the Most Common Triggers in Extrinsic Asthma?

If you are an extrinsic asthmatic, you have a great vulnerability to allergens. Therefore, you need to be aware of which allergens can trigger your immune system into defensive action.

Even though allergens are literally everywhere, they are sometimes avoidable. Allergens that you inhale are the most common triggers for extrinsic asthma. For an allergen to present a problem to a susceptible person, it must be abundant in the environment and have a transport system, such as wind currents, to carry it. Inhaled allergens vary greatly from place to place and present seasonal or perennial (year-round) problems, depending on their availability and nature.

Of the many possible offenders, the following are the most commonly recognized triggers of extrinsic asthma.

POLLENS

Pollen is a tiny, seedlike grain produced by plants, such as trees, grasses, and weeds. It is actually the living male germinal cell required for the fertilization and reproduction of its species. Pollen grains range in microscopic sizes, and are carried by insects and the wind. Wind-pollinated plants, called aeroallergens, present more problems for an extrinsic asthmatic than insect-pollinated plants. You can easily see the difference between these two types of plants. Wind-pollinated plants aren't nearly as attractive as those pollinated by insects because they don't have flowers that attract the insects. Since pollen is very buoyant, a gentle wind can carry it for miles, thereby producing high pollen concentrations in areas far from its original source.

Although pollen availability varies, depending on locality, in general there are three distinct pollinating seasons: early spring for trees, late spring and early summer for grasses, and late summer and fall (until the frost comes) for weeds. There is some overlapping of these seasons, though, because of the presence of small allergen particles, other than pollens, that are formed from the breakdown of plant materials and are found at times other than their normal pollen season.

Often we hear pollen counts given over the radio or television. A pollen count is a measurement of the density of the pollen in an air sample. Pollen counts vary a lot, but they can be used by an asthmatic as a rough guide to determine the possibility of individual allergy occurring in a certain location. For the long term, studying pollen counts can be important in predicting pollination patterns over a period of years. But for the short term, for the individual asthmatic, it holds less importance because it doesn't always correlate with exposure. This is because the pollen-count variability from one small area to the next depends on the pollen source and wind currents, as well as the type of pollen sampling method used. At any rate, it is interesting to know the pollen count in your area because it will give you a rough guide as to when to expect your asthma symptoms to get better or worse.

Tree Pollens   Wind-pollinated trees are a much greater source of allergy than insect-pollinated ornamental and fruit trees. Tree pollination occurs before, during, and shortly after the leaves develop in deciduous trees

(trees that lose their leaves in the fall). Some wind-pollinated trees guilty of producing asthma symptoms are oak, walnut, hickory, alder, birch, sycamore, ash, poplar, and cottonwoods.

Two common trees in the United States, the maple and the willow, create only a mild allergy problem because their pollen is mostly insect-pollinated. Another group of trees—known as conifers, or evergreens—produces so much pollen, it can be visible as a cloud in the air, and after settling, can change the color of the ground below. But these trees are rarely a source of allergy because their pollen is large and the outer shell of the pollen doesn't easily break down to expose the allergen. One of the few evergreens to cause allergy problems is mountain cedar. This compact tree, found from the hills of western Texas to the mountains of central Mexico, sheds pollen heavily from late December to February.

Tree pollens differ from each other, so if you're allergic to one tree, you are not necessarily allergic to other trees.

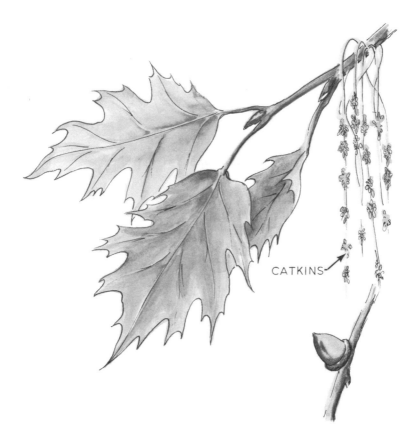

CATKINS

Red oak is a common source of tree pollen. The pollen comes from catkins, which appear before the leaves bud.

Grass Pollens   Grass pollen is a great enemy to extrinsic asthmatics in the United States. For frequency and severity of allergy symptoms, grass pollen ranks second only to ragweed in the United States, whereas it is the number one allergen in most other parts of the world. The blue grasses, Timothy (used to make hay), orchard grass, and redtop are among the most allergy-provoking grasses in southern Canada and the northeast two-thirds of the United States. In the southern part of the United States, major allergy sources are Bermuda, Bahia, and Johnson grasses.

Most of the allergenic grasses are cultivated; therefore, they abound

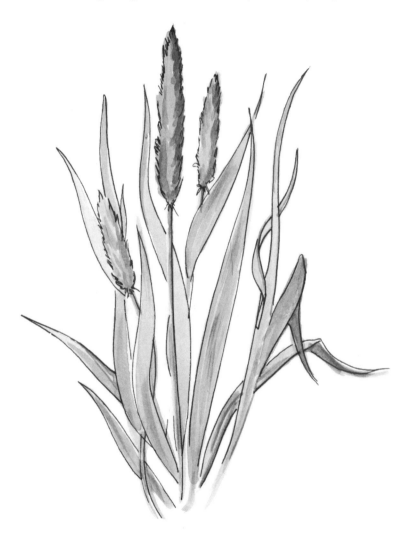

Timothy is a major source of grass pollen throughout the world. Its pollen comes from the catkins at the top of the plant.

where people live. In America, grass-pollen patterns are seasonal in the north and perennial in the south. The farther south you go and the warmer the climate, the longer the grass season. Coincidentally, at the time of grass pollination, the fertilized eggs (not pollen) from cottonwood and poplar trees become buoyant and resemble soft, cottonlike tufts; many asthmatics mistakenly attribute their symptoms to these floating balls of cotton when actually their allergy is due to grass pollen. Most grass pollens are similar, so if you're allergic to one, you're allergic to all (except for the pollen from Bermuda, Bahia, and Johnson grasses, which are different). Often grass pollination coincides with oak-tree pollination at the end of the spring, so that it becomes a time of double jeopardy for extrinsic asthmatics!

Weed Pollens   Weeds are plants that seem to grow anywhere people do not want them to grow. They have little or no agricultural or decorative value. From an allergy point of view, the most annoying weed is ragweed, the number one cause of allergy in the United States. It is estimated that a single ragweed plant may expel a million pollen grains in a single day, and that a square mile of ragweed plant produces 16 tons of pollen. Because of its buoyancy, ragweed really moves! Its pollen has been found as high as 14,000 feet in altitude and as far as 400 miles out at sea.

In North America, the central plains and eastern agricultural regions have the greatest concentrations of ragweed pollen. Ragweed grows better on land that's been cleared, and because it's an especially tough plant, it has taken over in many of these areas. Also, the long, hot autumns in the central plains and eastern agricultural regions are perfect for the growth of ragweed plants.

Although there are many different kinds of ragweed, the two most productive sources of ragweed pollen are the short and the giant (which may grow as high as 15 feet) ragweed plants. Both types grow from the Atlantic coast westwards, but they are especially prevalent in the Midwest. They don't exist in the Pacific Northwest nor in most of Europe.

Many other weeds besides ragweed cause allergy problems—such as cannabis (marijuana), burweed, cocklebur, lamb's quarter, pigweed, plantain, Russian thistle (tumbleweed), kochia (burning bush), sage, and western water hemp. Their pollination times don't always coincide with the ragweed season. Some will pollinate during the grass season, or between the grass and ragweed seasons. Airborne weed pollens leave the air with the first killing frost, which usually results in immediate relief of symptoms for anyone allergic to weeds.

During the ragweed and grass pollinating seasons, many asthmatics

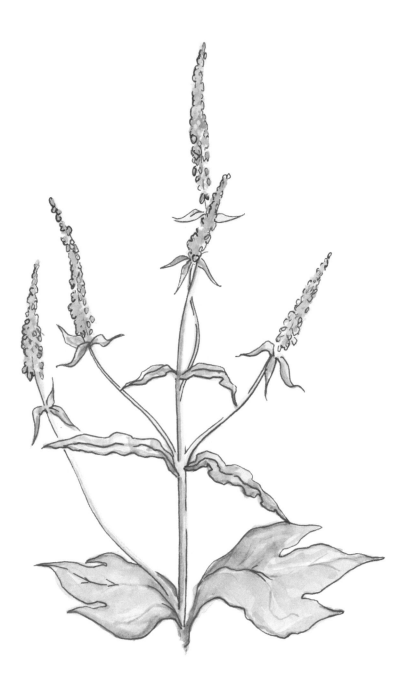

Ragweed is a major source of weed pollen in the midwestern part of the United States. The pollen comes from the catkins at the top of the plant.

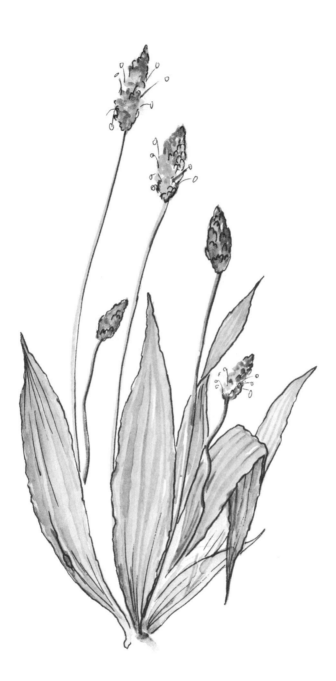

Plantain frequently grows in poorly maintained lawns, and is a common source of weed pollen.

mistakenly blame their symptoms on the flowering plants that bloom at the same times (in the Midwest, goldenrod blooms when ragweed pollinates, and roses bloom when grass pollinates; in the Northwest, Scotch broom blossoms when grass pollinates). But remember, the real culprits are not the pretty bloomers, but the less aesthetic wind-pollinated weeds mentioned earlier. (For more detailed information about pollens and their sources, turn to Appendix B.)

MOULDS

Moulds are among the most successfully adapted organisms on earth, and they present nothing but problems for the asthmatic. They exist in large numbers in nearly every environment—dry areas virtually devoid of water or other life, and moist areas with wide temperature extremes; they also exist in soil, fresh water, and salt water. Since they're so prolific, human exposure to them is unavoidable, regardless of the geographic region. Moulds are hardy parasites that produce spores, sort of one-celled "eggs" about the size of pollen grains, which are buoyant and airborne. These spores are the real culprits that wreak havoc on an allergic asthmatic. Airborne spores travel easily through our homes, especially with the prominence of forced-air heating systems. The small airborne particles permeate our furniture, drapes, and bedding, and they become a part of the general dust in our homes.

A home is a haven for moulds. Mould growth is so common in homes that it presents problems that are fairly difficult to avoid. Moulds growing in the home are referred to as "storage moulds." As the name indicates, storage moulds are the cause of rot and decay in grain, fruits, and vegetables. (Does this create a familiar picture?) You can see high concentrations of storage moulds in your home in dark places with high humidity because of the condensation of water on cool surfaces. High humidity is frequently found in bathrooms and basements, as well as refrigerator drip trays, garbage pails, and window ledges. Often, articles you've stored in damp, dark areas, such as the basement, will grow a green mould, called penicillium. Other allergenic moulds you may have in your home can exist in uncovered crawl spaces, soiled upholstery, shower curtains, attics, storage closets, air-conditioning systems, humidifiers, vaporizers, the soil of house plants, and house dust. See why we say indoor moulds are tough enemies to conquer?

Outdoor moulds are commonly called field moulds. They thrive on the field, on leaf piles, and on rotting, decaying wood. When soil is tilled or when leaves are disturbed, their spores are released in multitudes. The amount of spores derived from field moulds is much greater than the amount derived from storage moulds. And, at times, field moulds can equal or exceed the amount of ragweed pollen in an area. Mainly seasonal (from spring to late fall), field moulds diminish a bit with the first hard frost, but they don't actually disappear until several days after a very hard freeze. If you are an extrinsic asthmatic allergic to moulds, your symptoms may persist well into the winter months until a long, deep freeze occurs, ending the scourge of the mould spores. (For more information about moulds that commonly trigger asthma, turn to Appendix C.)

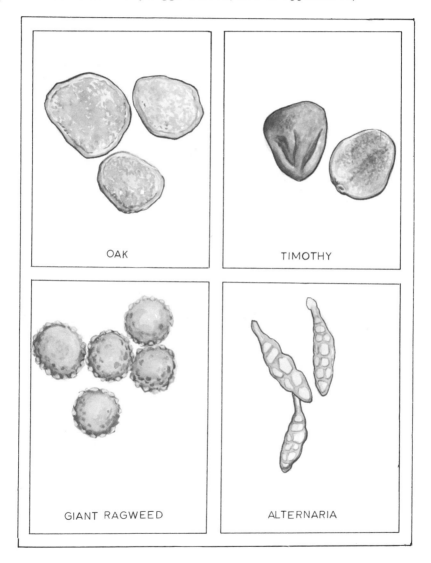

Common allergens are oak, Timothy, and giant ragweed pollens, and alternaria mould.

HOUSE DUST

Dust, as you well know, is everywhere, but did you know that it is a perfect transport system for other allergens? You may be surprised to find out that house dust is composed of organic and inorganic substances—such as animal dander, human skin and hair, plant fibres, clothing fibres, rotting food remains, insect parts, and last but most important, the dust mite. Although all of these substances together contribute to the allergic composition of house dust, it is the villainous dust mite that is probably the major allergen in house dust.

Dust mites are minuscule living organisms, which feed on human skin particles that are shed naturally. You can't see dust mites without the help

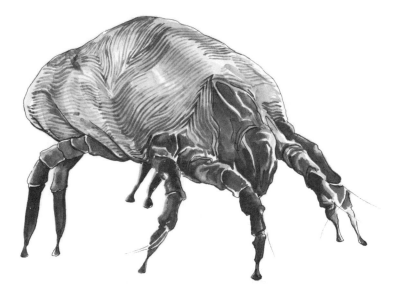

This is a drawing of a dust mite. This minuscule living organism is the major allergen in house dust.

of some powerful magnification, but they exist in great abundance in your home, especially on your mattress and the carpeted area around your bed. An estimated 42,000 mites exist in an ounce of mattress dust. The warm, humid environments of most homes are thriving grounds for these creatures. The dust-mite content of house dust varies, depending on the geographic area; for instance, dust mites are not found in dry regions or in high-altitude areas because these locations aren't moist enough for their growth.

Don't confuse house dust with the sooty dirt you see outdoors; for an asthmatic, outdoor dirt is irritating if inhaled, but house dust is allergenic and can set your symptoms into high gear. If your asthma is triggered by house dust, it may bother you year-round, with your symptoms becoming worse in the fall and winter when your house is closed up, the furnace is on, and dust is everywhere.

ANIMAL DANDERS

Those lovable, domestic pets that provide us with comfort and companionship are also prime prospects for triggering asthma symptoms. The allergic problem comes from the animal's dander, saliva, and urine—not from animal hair, as most people believe. Dander is shed by all living animals and it is always potentially allergenic. Processed furs, seen in coats and jackets, don't cause allergy because they are not living and do not shed dander. The most frequent troublemakers for allergic asthmatics are cats, dogs, hamsters, gerbils, and rabbits. Some farm animals—such as horses, hogs, cattle, and goats—can cause problems, too. Rats can be an allergen for people working in research.

COCKROACHES

Cockroaches have been around for a long time; they are among the oldest and most primitive of insects. In fact, some kinds of cockroaches have been associated so long with human beings that they may be said to be domesticated!

Cockroaches lay eggs in cases, cartons, and boxes in food-producing and food-storage warehouses. After you purchase food, you carry the eggs into your home inconspicuously, where they later hatch. Cockroaches can also enter your home through sewer systems, doorways, or cracks in the walls.

Cockroaches hide during the day in dark places and come out in search of food at night. Their allergen seems to be a major cause of asthma in many people. In fact, 50 to 70 percent of the asthmatic children and adults in two studies had asthmatic symptoms after being exposed to cockroaches. You can be exposed to cockroaches year-round, but your exposure may be greater during the winter, when they are more frequently found in the house.

INSECT PARTICLES

Inhaling insect particles can cause asthma. Insect allergens come from the particles that have broken down from insects. Two especially allergenic insects are the caddis fly and the mayfly. Caddis flies, found around the east end of Lake Erie, are abundant from June to late August. Caddis flies have small hairs covering their bodies, which break off and become wind-borne; these hairs are the source of allergy. Mayflies, found around the west end of Lake Erie, appear in June or July. They live only a few hours and shed a fragile outer skin. The debris from this skin produces sufficient airborne allergens to cause problems for you if you are an allergic asthmatic.

MISCELLANEOUS ALLERGENS

This category includes plant fibres—such as cottonseed, kapok, and flax-seed—that are widely used in consumer goods. These allergens are used for stuffing pillows, furniture, sleeping bags, and stuffed animals. They are used in cattle and poultry feed, as well.

Also included in this category is pyrethrum, which comes from pyre-thrum flowers, and is similar to the ragweed plant. It is used as an insecticide. If you are allergic to ragweed, you may notice a flare-up of symptoms when you are near an area that has been sprayed with pyre-thrum.

Another allergic annoyance for you can be feathers, which are often found in quilts, jackets, and sleeping bags, in addition to some beddings and pillows. Unfortunately, the processing of feathers for pillow stuffing doesn't remove the portions responsible for allergies.

Jute, used as backing on some rugs and in macramé materials, is another allergen for some allergic asthmatics.

FOODS

Although it's true that certain foods have been known to cause asthma, the subject of food allergy is open to controversy. Some adverse food reactions are allergic and some are not. For the reaction to be allergic, it must have an immunological basis; the IgE antibody must interact with the offending food and start the chain reaction that results in allergic symptoms. (If you have an adverse reaction that is not allergic in nature, you would have what is known as a *food intolerance*.)

According to findings recently released by the National Institutes of Health in the United States, food allergies causing asthma are not as common as people think. Nonetheless, a true allergic reaction to food can happen occasionally, and the allergic reaction usually occurs within one hour after eating. Food-allergy-induced asthma is most common in youngsters. If a food triggers your asthma, you'll probably have other symptoms—such as swelling around the eyes and nasal congestion, hives, and abdominal cramps. The most common food culprits are eggs, nuts, legumes (beans, peas, and peanuts), cottonseed, and seafood. (For a rundown on food families, refer to Appendix D.)

Recently, a growing number of asthmatics in the United States have been experiencing severe adverse reactions to foods treated with sulfites. Sulfites are used as preservatives and they keep foods looking fresh. We've had an increased exposure to sulfites in recent years with the booming popularity of salad bars (which until 1986 used sulfites) and with the growing tendency of the American public to eat in restaurants (a typical restaurant meal prior to 1986 could have contained 100 milligrams, or more, of sulfites). As a result of an increasing amount of asthma symptoms occurring in restaurant patrons sensitive to sulfites, in 1986 the United States Food and Drug Administration banned the use of sulfites on fresh fruits and vegetables in both restaurants and markets. (Sulfites have never been used on meat products or fish, other than shellfish.) Their use in other foods is still allowed, although it's presently being studied. Furthermore, the FDA is requiring the labelling of foods that contain relatively high amounts of sulfites. These foods are:

- all types of foods containing potato or potato products;
- dried fruits and vegetables;
- chilli mixes, hashes, chowders, and some tomato sauces; and
- syrups, toppings, some potted cheeses, cheese mixes, cheese paste, fruit juices, soft drinks, beer, wine, cider, vinegar, and pickles.

On labels, look for sulfite agents appearing under these names:

- potassium or sodium bisulfite,
- potassium or sodium metabisulfite,
- sodium sulfite, and
- sulfur dioxide.

The estimated frequency of sulfites causing asthma is about 3 to 5 percent. No one is sure how sulfites cause asthma, but it is known not to be caused through an allergic mechanism. Sulfites seem to cause asthma in some people because of an enzyme deficiency that has to do with their bodies' metabolism of sulfites.

DRUGS

An allergic drug reaction can cause asthma, but many adverse reactions to drugs are not true allergic reactions. Only those reactions that involve immune mechanisms are considered allergic. Drug allergies can occur with low dosages of a drug, and they usually occur after more than one exposure to the drug.

The most common drug producing a true allergic reaction is penicillin.

Often people allergic to the mould spore penicillium are mistakenly thought to be allergic to the penicillin drug, but there is actually no association between the two, even though the penicillin drug is extracted from penicillium mould.

o   o   o

Recognizing allergic triggers and learning how your body sets off an allergic response are positive steps you can take to further increase your understanding of asthma. However, it is important to realize that not *all* of the triggers discussed in this chapter will cause asthma symptoms in everyone. We are all unique individuals, and each of us needs to know which triggers are particular dangers for us to avoid. Furthermore, as we will see in the next chapter on intrinsic asthma, there are other nonallergic triggers that can provoke an asthmatic response in the extrinsic asthmatic. Knowing the facts is essential in coping with asthma, and will be the starting point from which you will eventually learn how to control it.

3

Understanding Intrinsic (Nonallergic) Asthma

Intrinsic asthma, otherwise known as nonallergic asthma, is not caused or triggered by allergies. People with intrinsic asthma have hyperreactive airways that overreact to a variety of nonallergic stimuli. Intrinsic asthma is triggered by viral infections, inhalation of irritating substances, stressful situations, exercise, and the effects of environmental factors such as weather and air pollution.

The onset of intrinsic asthma most frequently begins before the age of 3 or after the age of 30, although it's not uncommon to have an onset at any age.

In this chapter, we will learn about the causes of intrinsic asthma, the similarities and differences between intrinsic and extrinsic asthma, and the common nonallergic triggers for asthma.

What Are the Similarities Between Intrinsic and Extrinsic Asthma?

Whether your asthma is intrinsic or extrinsic, your symptoms will generally be the same. When you're exposed to a trigger, you may experience chest tightness, difficulty breathing, wheezing, and coughing. What happens inside the chest during an asthma attack is the same with intrinsic and extrinsic asthma: bronchospasm, production of excess mucus, and inflammation and swelling of the mucous membrane lining the bronchial tubes.

The real common denominator among all asthmatics, regardless of the type of asthma, is hyperreactive airways, or "twitchy airways," which means that the airways overreact and abnormally constrict after exposure to one or more triggering factors. Oversensitive airways are thought to be due to an imbalance in the body chemicals that regulate the opening and closing of the bronchial tubes. The chemicals responsible for keeping the airways open are blocked, making the airways hypersensitive and "twitchy" to both allergic and nonallergic triggers. A malfunction of the autonomic nervous system is in part responsible for this chemical imbalance.

What Are the Differences Between Intrinsic and Extrinsic Asthma?

The basic differences between the two kinds of asthma are the triggers that cause the asthma and the mechanisms used by our bodies to set off the asthmatic response. Intrinsic asthmatics are not allergic to inhaled allergens and do not have specific allergic IgE antibodies; they do not have asthma that is set off by an allergic trigger. Rather, the intrinsic asthmatic is only set off by nonallergic triggers, which have a direct effect on their oversensitive airways.

Along with the triggering factors and the mechanisms of response, the two types of asthma differ with regard to the usual age of onset; symptom patterns; history of allergic disease; skin-test response; eosinophilia (an increase in eosinophils, a type of white blood cell); serum IgE; response to immunotherapy (allergy shots); response to environmental avoidance of allergens; associated nasal, sinus, and skin conditions; and prognosis (prospect of recovery).

As we have already mentioned, the most frequent age of onset for intrinsic asthma is usually under 3 years, or over 30. Although the years between ages 3 and 30 are more common for the onset of extrinsic asthma, an intrinsic onset during these years is not uncommon. An intrinsic asthmatic's symptoms are more perennial and tend to be chronic, as opposed to the often seasonal symptoms experienced by the extrinsic asthmatic. Intrinsic asthma patterns are unpredictable and fluctuant, and tend to be worse in winter due to an increased incidence in respiratory infections, a major trigger for asthma.

Intrinsic asthmatics usually have no significant past personal or family history of *allergy*, whereas extrinsic asthmatics have a strong allergic family history. Intrinsic asthmatics and extrinsic asthmatics *both* have a high family history of *asthma*.

In terms of skin tests for allergies, intrinsic asthmatics generally have negative reactions, whereas the reactions of extrinsic asthmatics are positive.

Intrinsic asthmatics usually have a high eosinophil count in their blood and in their mucus; extrinsic asthmatics have a somewhat lower eosinophil count in these body fluids. Additionally, intrinsic asthmatics have a normal serum IgE antibody level, in contrast to the usually high level found in extrinsic asthmatics.

In terms of response to therapy and environmental control, the intrinsic asthmatic responds well to drugs, has some response to environmental control measures, and does not respond to immunotherapy (allergy shots). In contrast, the extrinsic asthmatic usually responds well to drugs, environmental control, and immunotherapy.

Often extrinsic asthmatics have hay fever and atopic dermatitis (eczema) associated with their asthma. Sometimes intrinsic asthmatics have nasal polyps and nasal congestion, sinusitis (inflammation of the sinuses), and/or aspirin sensitivity associated with theirs; when these three conditions are all present, the individual is said to have the "asthma triad."

Aspirin-sensitive asthmatics are also sensitive to nonsteroidal anti-inflammatory drugs because they are similar in their drug action. Aspirin-sensitive asthmatics have been suspected of being sensitive to tartrazine (a food additive and dye, commonly called FD&C Yellow #5), but this has been by and large overstated. Sensitivity to tartrazine is controversial.

The asthmatic who has aspirin sensitivity should avoid using aspirin, aspirin-containing products, and nonsteroidal anti-inflammatory drugs. Aspirin is present in many over-the-counter (O.T.C.) and prescription analgesics. It is also found in many common cold remedies. Aspirin is generally listed on the ingredient table as *acetylsalicylic acid*. If you suspect that you may be aspirin-sensitive, read the labels on all O.T.C. drugs carefully before you use them, and talk to your doctor about your possible sensitivity so that he may prescribe appropriate substitutions.

Salicylate, an ingredient in many foods and drugs, is chemically different from aspirin (acetylsalicylic acid) and doesn't cause the same asthmatic difficulties as aspirin. Usually foods and drugs containing salicylate—not acetylsalicylic acid—can be taken by an aspirin-sensitive asthmatic.

As for prognosis, children with intrinsic asthma often develop remissions as they grow older; however, approximately 25 percent will experience a recurrence of asthma in adulthood (recurrence is more common in women than in men). Intrinsic asthmatics who only get asthma attacks triggered by upper-respiratory infections are more likely to develop long-term remissions as they get older. Although adult intrinsic asthmatics have few permanent remissions, they do experience frequent short-term remissions. Some have no remissions, but their asthma can be controlled reasonably well with medication. Extrinsic asthmatics seem to become less symptomatic as they grow older, and their remission rate and/or cure rate can be significantly improved with allergic treatment.

Comparison of Extrinsic and Intrinsic Asthma

	Extrinsic Asthma (Allergic)	Intrinsic Asthma (Nonallergic)
Age of onset	3–30	Under 3, over 30 (sometimes in between)
Symptom patterns	Seasonal and/or perennial, often worse in spring and fall	Unpredictable fluctuations, often worse in winter
Family history of allergy	Yes	No
Family history of asthma	Yes	Yes
Skin tests	Positive	Negative
Eosinophil (a type of white blood cell) count	Variable, normal to high-normal range	High
Serum IgE (allergic antibody)	High or normal	Normal
Response to therapy and environmental avoidance of allergens	Good response to allergy shots and drugs, good response to environmental avoidance of allergens	Does not respond to allergy shots, good response to drugs, no response to environmental avoidance of allergens
Associated conditions	Atopic dermatitis (eczema), hay fever	Sinusitis, nasal polyps and nasal congestion, aspirin sensitivity
Prognosis	Good, less symptomatic with age, high remission rate with proper treatment	Remission rate high in children, especially if viral infection is only trigger; remission less common in adults

What Are the Most Common Triggers for Intrinsic Asthma?

As we have already discussed, it is important for an asthmatic to recognize the factors that can trigger an asthma episode. Remember that with intrinsic asthma, symptoms are not triggered by allergies, but only by nonallergic factors. (However, those factors that trigger intrinsic asthma can trigger extrinsic asthma also.)

Common nonallergic asthma triggers are irritating substances, infection, stress, exercise, and environmental factors including weather and air pollution.

IRRITATING SUBSTANCES

When irritating substances are present in the air, they cause windpipe irritation, which, in turn, provokes asthma symptoms. Actually, these substances are potential irritants to most people, but an asthmatic's hypersensitive airways exaggerate the problem. A common irritant that is only mildly annoying to most people can evoke severe symptoms in an asthmatic.

Therefore, asthmatics should beware of the following possible agitators: tobacco smoke, which is one of the major irritants; any substances that are easily vaporized and can directly irritate the windpipes, such as fumes and vapors from gasoline or diesel fuel, cleaning solvents, paints, paint thinner, and liquid-chlorine bleach; sprays from furniture polish, starch, cleaners, room deodorizers, deodorants, and perfumes, as well as hair sprays; talcum powders and scented cosmetics; and fumes from cooking odors—especially fish and animal odors. Also, the pine odor emitted from Christmas trees sometimes triggers flare-ups for certain asthmatics during the holiday season. In addition, the odor from raw cedar wood can trigger an asthma episode in a susceptible asthmatic.

INFECTION

Viral infections, such as colds and flu, are notorious asthma triggers; in fact, they are the primary provokers of intrinsic asthma. Furthermore, they frequently usher in the first onset of asthma. What may start as a simple cold may progress to a full-blown asthma attack because a viral infection makes the airways more sensitive and spastic. The increased airway reactivity may last up to 8 weeks following the initial viral infection. So, after the infection is over, chronic asthma may continue, with the airways even more reactive than before to additional viral infections and other asthma triggers. The respiratory viruses that most frequently trigger asthma are the common cold and flu viruses. Viruses damage the lining of the airways and therefore stimulate sensory nerve fibres, resulting in "reflex bronchospasm" of the windpipes; they also increase permeability of the airway mucous membrane for other irritants and allergens triggering asthma. In addition, a virus increases the chemical imbalance in an asthmatic, which results in increased bronchial sensitivity, chemical mediator release, and airway inflammation. Recurrent viral infections reinforce and maintain an asthmatic's airway hyperreactivity.

Bacterial infections play less of a role in triggering asthma than viral infections, but they *can* complicate the asthmatic condition. Bacterial infections are usually manifested in the form of sinusitis and pneumonia, which are two major conditions associated with asthma. Sinusitis frequently results in coughing attacks, which can be confused with asthma. However, the coughing attacks can also provoke an asthma attack.

STRESS

Emotional stress is a part of everyday life to a greater or lesser degree. Emotions affect both our psychological and physical well-being. When we experience stress, our adrenaline flows, our heart pounds, our breath comes faster, and our muscles get tense. Our response to stress may stem from such strong emotions as fear, anxiety, frustration, or anger. Certainly, responses to stress can have an effect on anyone's breathing, but the asthmatic is particularly vulnerable. When you're tense, the smooth, relaxed functioning of your airways can be disrupted. Consequently, it is not difficult to calculate the degree to which stress can affect your asthma.

It is important to recognize that while emotions don't actually cause asthma, they can certainly increase or decrease the frequency and severity of your attacks. (We deal further with the topic of stress and its relationship to asthma in Chapter 15.)

EXERCISE

Some people develop asthmatic reactions during or following exercise or exertion. Exercise forces the lungs to work more quickly and to exchange air more rapidly. When exercising or during times of physical exertion, breathing deeply can possibly stimulate the asthmatic's "twitchy" airways and thus provoke an attack. This occurs because of a loss of moisture from the airways, resulting in an increased salt content (osmolality). This, in turn, stimulates the release of various chemical mediators, resulting in an asthma attack. (We address the subject of asthma triggered by exercise more comprehensively in Chapter 13.)

ENVIRONMENTAL FACTORS

Weather   Weather is the result of multiple meteorological factors, including temperature, wind velocity, barometric pressure, and humidity. The influence that weather has on producing asthma symptoms is indefinite and open to controversy. It is unclear if weather factors per se precipitate asthmatic symptoms or if weather factors act by virtue of environmental modifications to bring about asthmatic symptoms. For example, weather can affect asthma because of its effect on dispersion or retention of air pollution. It even affects extrinsic asthma because local vegetation as well as pollen-and-spore-dispersion patterns are influenced by seasonal weather conditions. Indeed, weather changes may affect the concentration of all air particles in a geographical location; it is common knowledge that air inversions, characterized by periods of air stagnation, cause an increase in air pollution, and are associated with an increase in respiratory problems.

The best thing for you to do is to become aware of the effects the weather can have on your asthma. Here are some general observations related to the weather and its effects on asthma:

- Cold, dry air seems to present problems for asthmatics. It is possible that asthma triggered by cold, dry air is due to the stimulation of the upper-airway nerve receptors, causing "reflex bronchospasm." Or perhaps it's due to a mechanism that's similar to that found in exercise-induced asthma—the release of chemical mediators because of an increased salt content from drying of the airways.

- High-humidity readings are associated with increased asthma symptoms. During times of high humidity, some people experience hyperventilation (breathing in and out more air than they need, while at the same time experiencing the feeling of not getting enough air). Hyperventilation may be confused with and/or trigger asthma. Likewise, changes in barometric pressure sometimes can cause problems for the asthmatic.

- Wind can blow smog and air pollution away, but it can also bring pollen directly to an asthmatic. In addition, low wind velocity and temperature inversions can increase an asthmatic's exposure to smog.

- Rain can diminish allergens, irritants, and pollutants. But rainy, humid weather conditions are also great for facilitating vegetation and mould growth, which results in a greater release of pollen and mould spores later.

From this list, you can see that weather factors can play a significant role in potentially creating problems for the asthmatic.

Air Pollution   Another common problem for the asthmatic is air pollution, which is an atmospheric accumulation of substances, usually man-made, to a degree that becomes injurious to humans, animals, and plants. Air pollution is associated with two kinds of smog: *industrial smog* and *photochemical smog*. These two are by no means mutually exclusive; in fact, frequently both are present in a given area at the same time.

Industrial smog is predominant in large industrial cities, and is the result of the combustion of solid or liquid fossil fuels. The main contaminants of industrial smog are sulfur dioxide, sulfuric acid, and atmospheric particulate matter.

When sulfur dioxide combines with water in the atmosphere, it eventually becomes sulfuric acid. Sulfuric acid is more irritating than sulfur dioxide, and also may be formed when sulfur dioxide comes in contact with the water in the mucus on the surface of our airways. This can trigger asthma.

Atmospheric particles include both liquid and solid particles that may originate from such sources as smoke, dust, soot, and chemical fumes. These pollutants can cause direct, adverse effects on our airways.

Photochemical smog occurs mostly in cities with a high density of automobiles and adequate sunlight to permit photochemical reactions. The reaction of sunlight and heat on automobile exhaust fumes results in the formation of ozone, nitrogen dioxide, and other oxide chemicals, which contaminate the air.

Ozone is the main component of photochemical smog, sometimes making up as much as 90 percent of it. During an episode of heavy smog, its concentration can reach very high levels. Ozone can directly trigger asthma.

Nitrogen dioxide is found in urban atmospheres since its main source is automobile exhaust fumes. Nitrogen dioxide may react with the water in the mucus on the surface of our airways to form nitric acid, which triggers asthma.

While both air pollution and weather factors have an effect on asthma, it is often the interrelationship between the two that ultimately affects the asthmatic.

In addition to knowing what kind of asthma you have and how your body sets off the asthmatic response, one of the most important steps you can take in controlling your asthma is to know what causes it. Our environment and our lives are full of potential asthma triggers. It's important for you to be able to recognize them, know their dangers, and understand how they can affect your asthma. Then you can begin to work as a teammate with your doctor in both preventing and controlling your asthma.

o   o   o

As we end this chapter on intrinsic asthma, we want to emphasize that many asthmatics are not purely "intrinsic" or "extrinsic," but a combination of the two. Hence, their treatment and course will not fall clearly into one group or the other, but will overlap into elements of both. We have separated asthma into intrinsic and extrinsic categories mainly for the sake of clarity.

4

Understanding Asthma in Children

Your child is sick again. And once again, those familiar feelings of frustration, anxiety, and resentment settle in you and then you feel guilty. After all, your child is ill and needs you. You dislike being a pessimist, but every time he gets a cold you just know it will end in disaster—sleepless nights for both of you, coupled with his constant coughing and wheezing and your efforts at easing his discomfort while you try to hush your own growing fears. Tomorrow there will be another trip to the doctor, which will result in the diagnosis you've come to expect: "bronchitis" or "pneumonia." On the way home from the doctor's office, you'll need to stop off at the pharmacy for yet another prescription of antibiotics. You've done this so many times, you could probably do it with your eyes closed.

You do everything right to take care of your child, complying with your doctor's method of treatment. You want to have faith, but you only feel discouragement. In spite of your conscientious care, your child still gets colds—and he coughs and can't breathe. What is wrong? How come you're doing everything right and your child *still* keeps getting so sick? The answer may be that your child has asthma.

Interesting Facts and Statistics about Childhood Asthma

1. Asthma is the most common of all lung diseases of childhood.

2. Approximately 50 percent of the estimated 10 million asthmatics in the United States are children.

3. Around 8 percent of all children experience problems with asthma.

4. Almost half of all asthma in adults begins in childhood.

5. Approximately half of all childhood asthma begins before age 3.

6. Until puberty, boys are affected twice as frequently as girls; this trend

reverses in the teens and early adulthood, with females becoming more affected than males in mid- to late adulthood.

7. Boys are not only more likely to develop asthma in childhood, but are more likely to have severe asthma.

8. Immunotherapy (allergy shots) tends to be more effective with children and young adults than with older adults.

9. When asthma develops during the first 2 decades of life, it's more likely to be related to allergies.

10. Children under 5 years old are at a greater risk of having severe asthma attacks that result in major complications or death.

11. Asthma is the number one cause of time loss from school due to chronic illness, accounting for about 25 percent of such absences.

12. For patients less than 17 years of age, asthma accounts for 33 percent of the visits they make to physicians for chronic disease.

Is Childhood Asthma the Same As Adult Asthma?

Asthma is asthma; its definition applies to any man, woman, or child who has the disease. Asthma is a condition of the bronchial tubes, characterized by episodes of constriction and increased mucous production. When people have asthma, their bronchial tubes are supersensitive to various stimuli, or triggers. Because of this sensitivity, their windpipes react far more than they should to triggers and produce asthma symptoms. (Hence, all people with asthma are said to have "twitchy airways.") This happens because of an improper functioning of some of the biochemical and neurological systems that regulate the amount of airway narrowing, which is caused by these triggers. Overreactivity of the bronchial tubes is the major feature separating the asthmatic from the nonasthmatic child or adult.

During an attack, all asthmatics experience common symptoms—such as chest tightness, difficulty inhaling and exhaling, production of large amounts of mucus in the windpipes, coughing, and wheezing. Asthma often begins after a cold or flu infection, or during a pollen or mould season; generally, it can be triggered by any viral infection or allergen. It can also be triggered by exercise, exposure to irritating substances, stress, and weather changes. As with adults, some children can be symptom-free between attacks, whereas others seem to have some degree of symptoms present all the time. With children, however, symptoms can develop more quickly and can be more severe. This happens because their smaller airways can close more quickly and produce more mucus that easily accumulates and obstructs their tiny airways. It is important to note that not *all* asthmatic symptoms need be present for one to experience an asthma attack. For instance, not all asthmatics wheeze. And sometimes wheezing is so slight, it can only be heard with a stethoscope. With some asthmatics, coughing is the only symptom present. Asthmatic symptoms may vary throughout the day, often becoming more noticeable at night.

Children and adults can have either extrinsic (allergic) or intrinsic (nonallergic) asthma, or both. While their symptoms are generally the same, intrinsic and extrinsic asthmatics differ in what triggers their asthma and in what mechanisms their bodies use to set off the asthmatic response.

Adults and children *aren't* the same physically, emotionally, or socially, and the basic difference in the adult and child asthmatic lies therein. Children's bodies are still in various stages of development. Also, children have a different perception of themselves and their world than adults. Asthma can be a source of chronic fatigue for children, and may interfere with their sleep, school performance, family and peer interaction, normal exercise, and general physical development. In addition, it can drain the entire family's emotions and finances. Although hope looms on the horizon, asthma remains the leading chronic disease of childhood.

What Is the Usual Development and Course of Childhood Asthma?

For children, the severity and prognosis of asthma seem to be related to the age when the asthma begins and to the kind of asthma the child has. For example, if your child's asthma began before he was 6 months old, his prognosis may be worse in terms of severity and duration than if his asthma began later in childhood. If your child has severe asthma in his first few years of life, he will have less of a chance of long-term remission as he gets older. Children with less severe asthma at a young age have a better chance of it going away as they get older.

Intrinsic (nonallergic) asthmatics frequently become symptom-free later in childhood, but their asthma may recur in adulthood. Extrinsic (allergic) asthmatics may also improve with age, especially if their allergies are treated. In general, if the asthma (intrinsic or extrinsic) hasn't gone away by puberty, it's unlikely to ever go away completely. The old belief that "kids outgrow their asthma" isn't necessarily true.

The development and course of asthma is influenced by heredity. When both parents have asthma, there's a 50 percent chance of asthma occurring in their offspring; when one parent has it, a 25 percent chance. Parents with severe asthma are likely to have children with severe asthma. Children don't inherit asthma itself, but the *tendency* to develop it. However, sometimes even genetically identical twins differ in terms of the severity of their asthma, and occasionally one of them may not have asthma at all.

This is because other factors besides heredity—such as certain viral infections, exposure to allergens, and other environmental circumstances—can play a significant role in causing asthma.

Breast feeding in the first few months of life might lessen the child's risk of extrinsic asthma in later life, but data on this is inconclusive. Presently, breast feeding is a popular, but unproven, preventive measure for asthma.

No two children are identical in the way their asthma occurs. For many, the problem is "mild," with relatively few symptoms and only occasional flare-ups. For others, the problem is "severe," with the disease being the central problem in their lives and in the lives of their families. Asthma is medically classified as either mild, moderate, or severe, but its development and course can be as individual as the child who has it.

What constitutes mild, moderate, and severe asthma? The following table gives information on these classifications.

Severity Classifications of Childhood Asthma

Mild asthmatics	• have less than 6 mild attacks per year,
	• are symptom-free between attacks,
	• can function normally between attacks,
	• need no medication between attacks, and
	• require no hospitalizations.
Moderate asthmatics	• have 6 to 12 moderate attacks per year,
	• have mild to moderate symptoms between attacks,
	• have some difficulty functioning normally between attacks,
	• usually need medication between attacks to keep well,
	• occasionally need short periods of taking steroid medication, and
	• occasionally require hospitalization.
Severe asthmatics	• have more than 6 severe attacks per year despite continued medication,
	• have considerable difficulty functioning normally between attacks,
	• are often dependent on steroid medication for prolonged periods of time, and
	• require 2 or more hospitalizations per year.

Severe asthma resulting in death is infrequent in children. Nonetheless, children under age 5 are the ones at the greatest risk of death from severe asthma. This is because of their smaller airways that close more quickly and plug up with mucus more readily; also, children's complications with severe asthma are more difficult to treat and control. (See Chapter 11 for information on complications with asthma.)

What Are the Common Triggers of Asthma in Children?

Asthmatic triggers are factors that can bring about or set off asthma symptoms. Asthmatic triggers are the same in adults and children; however, there are certain triggers that play a more prevalent role in childhood asthma. These triggers are *viral respiratory infection, exercise,* and occasionally *food.* First we'll look at these common triggers for childhood asthma, and then at the full picture of asthmatic triggers that could be setting off your child's asthma.

VIRAL RESPIRATORY INFECTION

Viral respiratory infections are among the most common triggers of asthma in children. Viruses damage the lining of the airways, causing stimulation of nerve fibres, which results in windpipe spasms. Further, viruses increase the imbalance that asthmatics have in their autonomic nervous system, which controls the reactivity of their windpipes, and also increase chemical mediator release. In addition, viruses increase permeability of the airway mucous membrane for other irritants and allergens triggering asthma. Virally induced attacks usually last weeks, even if the virus infection disappears in a few days. Since young children have had little exposure to respiratory viruses, they have not yet developed immunity to viruses. Therefore, they may develop as many as six to twelve virally induced infections and related asthma attacks per year. This high attack rate can continue until they gradually develop immunity to the infectious agents. Then the frequency of asthma attacks often diminishes.

EXERCISE

Exercise and physical exertion can bring on asthma symptoms in an asthmatic child. It is particularly common in childhood for exercise to trigger asthma since children are spontaneously more active than adults; in fact, exercise triggers asthma in as much as 95 percent of all asthmatic children, and exercise may be the only trigger for asthma in some children. (The link between asthma and exercise is discussed in greater detail in Chapter 13.)

FOOD

While food allergies can produce gastrointestinal problems in children, they don't often cause asthma. When food does trigger asthma, it is usually in the early years of life and it is often associated with eczema and nasal allergies. Foods are more apt to trigger asthma in early infancy and childhood than in adulthood. As a child grows older, other allergies more commonly provoke asthma, and food allergies play a lesser role. The foods that most commonly provoke asthma in children are eggs, nuts, legumes (beans, peas, and peanuts), cottonseed, and seafood. Milk triggers asthma infrequently.

To help you get a clear picture of the triggers that most commonly set off asthma, we have separated them into extrinsic and intrinsic triggers in the "at-a-glance" table that follows. (For complete information on all of these triggers, refer to Chapters 2 and 3.) Remember, for children and adults alike, the differences between extrinsic and intrinsic asthma lie in the triggers that provoke an attack and the mechanisms their lungs use to set off the asthmatic response. However, the symptoms and what happens inside the chest during an attack are the same regardless of the kind of asthma.

Triggers in Childhood Asthma

Extrinsic Triggers* (Allergic)	Intrinsic Triggers** (Nonallergic)
• **Pollens:** trees, grasses, and weeds	• **Irritating substances:** any substance—such as smoke, odors, or vapors—whose presence in the air provokes asthma
• **Moulds:** found everywhere, both indoors and outdoors	
• **House dust:** a prevalent allergen, especially in the bedroom	• **Viral infection:** the #1 asthma provoker in children
• **Animal danders:** common allergens for children, especially from cats and dogs	• **Stress:** can greatly affect the frequency and severity of asthma attacks
• **Miscellaneous allergens:** such as feathers, kapok, jute, and other substances commonly found in our environment	• **Exercise:** plays a primary role in triggering asthma in children
• **Food:** infrequently triggers asthma, but when it does, it's usually in children under age 3	• **Environmental factors:** weather changes and air pollution

*For extrinsic asthmatics, food allergens that provoke asthma can be common in children under age 3, but they become less common as the children grow older. At about age 3, animal danders, dust, and moulds play a significant role because children at this age are frequently in the house, playing on the floor, where these allergens exist. From age 4 on, pollens begin to play an equal and then greater role as asthma-provoking allergens.
**These intrinsic triggers can provoke asthma symptoms in extrinsic asthmatics as well.

Once you know what triggers or combination of triggers are provoking your child's asthma and you understand why the asthma response occurs, you will be ready to work with your doctor to help control the condition. In upcoming chapters, we will discuss how to diagnose, treat, and control your child's asthma.

Does Childhood Asthma Affect the Growth and Development of Children?

Two major kinds of growth changes can result from asthma: chest deformities and height suppression.

Severe, chronic asthma in infancy and early childhood can cause chest deformity, which consists of an increased chest size (a barrel shape) because of overinflation of the lungs. This deformity can be reversed if asthma is controlled well.

Height suppression can occur with any severe, chronic disease—and asthma is no exception. Asthma has a greater adverse effect on height when it's severe and of early onset. (So you can see how important early diagnosis and treatment can be!) Often, suppressed growth related to asthma has been blamed on the use of steroids in treating the disease. But, when *properly prescribed and administered*, steroids do not alter growth patterns. Actually, growth complications related to asthma are due more to the chronic illness itself than to the drugs used to treat it.

What's the Association Between Asthma and Infections?

As we discussed earlier, viral infections—such as colds and flu—trigger asthma. Bacterial infections—such as sinusitis, pneumonia, and ear infections—seem to occur more frequently in asthmatic children, but only sinusitis is a trigger for asthma. Fever is a symptom of both viral and bacterial infections. When your child develops asthma in conjunction with a fever, it usually indicates that a viral infection—as opposed to a bacterial infection—is present. However, it's possible for a bacterial infection to be present, too.

If a fever persists longer than 3 days, you should see your doctor to determine whether the infection is viral or bacterial. Bacterial infections require antibiotics, whereas viral infections do not. You should also see your doctor if asthma symptoms aren't controlled by usual medications; he can determine whether additional medicine is needed to control the asthma symptoms.

What Can Happen If a Child's Asthma Is Not Controlled?

If asthma isn't controlled due to lack of medical attention, or because the condition wasn't recognized or the usual medication didn't work, it can progress to a severe state called status asthmaticus, which doesn't readily respond to medical treatment. It is asthma out of control. Status asthmaticus usually requires hospitalization, and can become life-threatening. (Read more about this severe state of asthma in Chapter 11.)

Can Asthma Cause Permanent Damage to a Child's Lungs and Heart?

Asthma almost never causes permanent damage to a child's lungs and heart. The changes that occur during an asthma attack—narrowing of the bronchial tubes, swelling of the membrane lining the bronchial tubes, and formation of mucous plugs in the bronchial tubes—are all reversible when asthma is brought under control. There doesn't appear to be any scarring or permanent lung damage caused by asthma.

Because of air trapping in the lungs, children with asthma can develop a barrel-shaped chest, resembling the chest often seen on adults with emphysema. But asthma doesn't evolve into emphysema. Asthma and emphysema are two distinct diseases that aren't related. (For more information on emphysema and other lung diseases, refer to Chapter 6.)

During an asthma attack, children usually have a rapid heartbeat due to low oxygen levels, the stress involved in labored breathing, and anxiety. Even the normal side effects of some of the commonly used asthma medications can increase a child's heartbeat. However, children generally tolerate the rapid heartbeat well and no permanent heart damage develops.

How Can You Tell If the Signs and Symptoms Indicate Asthma or Something Else?

Asthmatic symptoms are basically:
- difficulty inhaling and exhaling,
- general shortness of breath,
- feeling of chest tightness,
- coughing (loose or tight, dry or producing mucus), and
- wheezing (not always present).

Recognizing labored breathing problems in your child isn't too difficult. You know your child, and are attuned to his symptoms that signal difficulty. On occasion, diagnosing asthma can be tricky because breathing problems can be symptomatic of other ailments in children. In fact, many of these ailments can coexist with asthma.

It is often difficult to discriminate between asthma and other medical conditions that exhibit similar symptoms. However, the great majority of infants who have recurrent breathing problems usually have asthma.

When your child has wheezing and/or coughing attacks, asthma, rather than other causes, should be suspected if:

- there are recurrent episodes as opposed to a singular episode,
- there is a family history of allergy or asthma (especially in the parents), and
- there are frequent problems with nose and sinus congestion.

Other causes of breathing difficulties in children might be confused with asthma. Some of the most common ones are discussed below.

Aspirated Objects   Children can easily swallow any tiny object, which can become lodged in and obstruct their respiratory tract, resulting in coughing, wheezing, or choking. Unfortunately, symptoms may not arise immediately, and they may be variable, depending on the type of foreign object, the site where it is lodged, and the length of time it remains lodged. It's important to discuss this possibility with your doctor if you suspect it.

Croup (Laryngotracheobronchitis)   Croup usually occurs in children under 5 years old. It is characterized by a sudden nocturnal onset of a seallike barking cough, and hoarseness. Croup is a common condition, due to an ordinary respiratory flu or coldlike viral infection. In younger children, this results in inflammation of the larynx, trachea, and upper windpipes. However, in older children and adults, these viruses simply result in an upper-respiratory infection (the common cold). With croup, it is difficult for the child to get air *into* the lungs; with asthma, it is hard to get air *out* of the lungs. With croup, often a loud, harsh stridor is heard upon *inhaling*; with asthma, often wheezing is heard upon *exhaling*. In young children, croup and asthma can be confused because their symptoms are so similar. If your child has been diagnosed as having croup on two or more occasions, ask your doctor about the possibility of his having asthma.

Bronchitis (Bronchiolitis)   Asthma symptoms are frequently mistaken for bronchitis. As with asthma, bronchitis generally occurs in conjunction with an upper-respiratory infection. Your child may develop a dry, hacking cough, which will become loose and produce mucus a few days after it starts. Often wheezing occurs, and your child may experience a great deal of difficulty breathing, chest tightness, and a loss of appetite. A fever may be present. A single episode of bronchitis may simply be bronchitis. *But when your child keeps getting "bronchitis," he is likely to have asthma, especially if there is a family history of asthma.*

Acute Epiglottitis   Epiglottitis is an inflammation of the epiglottis, the small cap that closes off the trachea when you swallow. The onset is sudden. The child usually has a high fever and complains of a sore throat or of pain in the throat. Lethargy, difficulty breathing, and drooling are other symptoms. Acute epiglottitis is usually caused by a bacteria, and requires aggressive antibiotic treatment. It definitely warrants prompt medical attention because the swollen epiglottis may completely block off the trachea and cause suffocation.

Cystic Fibrosis   This is a genetically transmitted disease, which occurs almost exclusively in Caucasian children once in every 2,000 births. Cystic fibrosis is a progressive disease, usually involving the respiratory system, and is characterized by bronchial infections, coughing, wheezing, and poor growth. Symptoms may appear weeks or months after birth. Cystic fibrosis should be suspected in any child who has recurrent bronchial infections with the production of large amounts of thick mucus, who also has poor physical development. Cystic fibrosis is diagnosed by a simple measurement of sweat for chloride. However, a diagnosis of cystic fibrosis doesn't necessarily rule out asthma since the two conditions can coexist in a child.

If you question whether your child's symptoms are due to asthma, it is best to consult your doctor about the possibility. The sooner a correct diagnosis is made, the quicker your child's condition will be able to be controlled.

What Physical and Emotional Problems Do Children with Asthma Face?

Children with asthma face a variety of physical and emotional problems, which can have a tremendous impact on the quality of their lives. They must be able to deal with their asthma in a way that enables them to feel equal to their nonasthmatic peers. More importantly, they need to realize that they *can* control and cope with their asthma—and that once they learn how, they can do most of the things they want to do.

Let's look at some of the problems your child may encounter in living with asthma. We'll discuss the ways asthma can affect your child physically and emotionally, as well as intellectually.

PHYSICAL EFFECTS OF ASTHMA

Asthma has a variety of physical effects on children. The following are the major areas affected:

Activity   Asthmatic breathing requires more effort than nonasthmatic breathing. Asthma triggered by exercise may cause children to restrict the physical activities that are so important in their growing lives. However, asthma can be managed so that children are able to enjoy normal activities.

Posture   Habitual use of shoulder and neck muscles for breathing may lead a child to carry his shoulders in an up-and-forward fashion, which can cause a round-shouldered posture. Poor posture can create self-image problems. Children can be taught proper breathing techniques to mini-mize posture problems, which, in turn, will invariably have a positive effect on their self-image. (For information about breathing techniques, refer to Chapter 15.)

Growth   Although mild to moderate asthma usually doesn't affect growth, chronic, severe, or poorly controlled asthma may have a slowing effect on growth. Obviously, growth-suppression problems can lower a child's self-image and cause further coping problems. Proper treatment by a knowledgeable physician can make a difference in growth suppression and in the inherent problems it holds for your maturing child.

EMOTIONAL EFFECTS OF ASTHMA

Along with physical effects, asthma has some demonstrable effects on a child's emotional development and vice versa. The idea that the psyche, or mind, has an influence on asthma is now taken for granted. The mind and emotions intertwine, and have a direct bearing on an individual's ability to cope. Recent studies have strongly indicated that the coping styles of children and their families can intensify or lessen asthma.

An interesting story reported from the American Lung Association states that Theodore Roosevelt had asthma as a child, and that many authorities think his asthma was specifically related to an emotionally stressful home situation. It has been speculated that the improvement in his health when he left the East to live in Wyoming was due to his removal from the emotional stresses at home that provoked his asthma. Although this analysis was made years after his death, it appears that the relationship between asthma and the stresses in his life were not merely coincidental. In his case, it seems that relief of stress resulted in improvement of his asthma.

On the other hand, emotions are an individual's response to living, and any number of them may be experienced by your asthmatic child. The following are some of the most common emotions experienced by asthmatic children:

Anger and Resentment   Your child may feel angry and resentful that he must deal with asthma when other children around him don't have to. "Why do I have asthma?" "Why can't I run and play without having a hard time breathing?" "Why do I always have to take medicine?" Do these questions sound familiar? The feelings beneath them are real and normal for a child who just wants to experience living without all the consequences of having asthma.

Fear   Your asthmatic child may fear suffocation or death during an asthma attack. He may become anxiety ridden, worrying about having another attack. Periods of separation from your family, caused by hospitalizations, may cause your asthmatic child further worry and anxiety. Additional fears may arise if your child feels rejected by other children for being "different." As your child begins to understand and learn about asthma, his feelings of fear will lessen.

Inferiority   An inability to participate in various physical activities, poor scholastic performance due to absences from school, and generally feeling different from others can cause an asthmatic child to feel inferior. It's important for feelings of inferiority to be openly discussed among the physician, parents, and child. With good communication and understanding, the child can learn how to effectively deal with feelings of inferiority and eventually overcome them.

Depression   Not surprisingly, depression can settle in on your child as he tries to cope with having asthma. Coping is a big job, but it's not impossible to learn with your help. Encourage your child to discuss such feelings as depression, fear, and anger. By discussing these feelings, he will come to understand them better, and this will help him cope.

Clearly the emotional impact of having asthma may be more far reaching than the physical realities of the disease. The emotional impact, if not properly dealt with, can virtually ruin the joys of childhood. Only through education and understanding can we hope to help our children cope with and control their asthma, which will in turn ultimately enhance the quality of their lives. Education and understanding will also help them grow in healthy mental and physical states towards adulthood.

EFFECTS ON INTELLECTUAL DEVELOPMENT

Asthma can effect a child's intellectual development since it's a frequent cause of absenteeism from school. In addition, asthma medications can have some undesirable side effects, such as irritability and nervousness, which can affect a child's behavior and learning ability. Also, sometimes a child's attention span dwindles after taking medicine. Add all this to an inability to concentrate because of a poor night's sleep (from so much coughing) and you have some definite problems that interfere with the learning process. (For further details about asthma and school, see Chapter 12.)

Resources To Help You and Your Child Cope with Asthma

Over the past decade, a number of programs have evolved to help the asthmatic child and his family understand asthma and all its ramifications. Although these programs have goals that are similar to the goals of this book, they are presented in a format that specifically meets the needs of young children. These goals are:

- to give information about asthma to lessen fear and misunderstanding about the disease and to encourage the child's responsibility in playing a more active role in determining proper courses of treatment for his asthma;
- to train the asthmatic child in decision-making skills by teaching how and when to take medications, how and when to avoid specific triggers, when to ask for medical help, and how to function in various settings (school, sports, home);
- to teach the child and family how to cope with the consequences of asthma associated with stress, resulting from family, school, and social problems, or the asthma condition itself; and
- to teach the child breathing-relaxation techniques to enable him to help minimize some of the discomforts and stresses of asthma.

One example of an asthma educational program, which we helped develop and actively support, is the Huff and Puff Family Asthma Program, sponsored by St. John's Hospital in Springfield, Illinois. This program emphasizes education for asthmatic children and their families by using various educational formats, including puppets; creative dialogue and role playing; and stories and songs to teach children about their disease, medications, specific triggers, and ways to manage their condition. The program focuses on helping them eliminate the fear and stigma associated with asthma. Also, it teaches children breathing-relaxation techniques and allows them to identify, understand, and cope with the feelings of fear, anger, and frustration that are often associated with asthma. In addition, its informational lectures, videos, and group discussions help the parents to better understand their child's condition and to learn about ways in which they can help their child cope with asthma.

Other similar programs throughout the United States include: ACT program, developed at the University of California at Los Angeles (U.C.L.A.); Asthma Self-Management Program, developed at Columbia University (New York, New York); Captain Respirator, developed by the National Jewish Center (Denver, Colorado); a training program, developed by the American Institute of Research (Palo Alto, California); and a family asthma program, developed by Children's Hospital (Buffalo, New York).

For information on other available asthma-education programs in the United States, contact your local American Lung Association, local hospitals, or the American Academy of Allergy. (We have compiled a listing of summer camps for asthmatic children that is based on information from the American Lung Association—turn to Appendix F for this listing.) Taking part in a group educational experience can further enhance both your child's and your own coping skills.

Diagnosing Asthma in Adults and Children

5

A Visit to the Allergist— Diagnosing Asthma in Children and Adults

When you become aware that you or your child might have asthma, it would be a good idea to visit a specialist who diagnoses and treats asthma and allergic diseases. A doctor who specializes in this area is known as an allergist. Allergists have had special training in both pediatric and adult allergy and should be board-certified in allergy and immunology. Prior to training in allergy, they must have served a residency in pediatrics or internal medicine and become board-certified in either of these specialties.

There are several advantages in consulting an allergist. First of all, an allergist has had extensive training and experience in all allergic diseases, but especially in asthma. Being knowledgeable about all aspects of asthma, he will be aware of the best diagnostic techniques and treatment methods available for your condition. Also, an allergist will be able to guide you in your self-help efforts to control and cope with your asthma.

The best way to find a qualified allergist in your area is to ask your own physician to recommend one. Or you can discover names of qualified allergists on your own by contacting your local medical society. In the United States, another way to find a qualified allergist is to phone the American Academy of Allergy and Immunology.

You can "breathe easier" just knowing that with the right medical help, you'll be on the road to control or recovery. In this chapter, we'll discuss what you may typically experience on your visit to the allergist (both adults and children are generally diagnosed by the same techniques).

What Can I Do To Prepare for My Visit to an Allergist?

Basically, the best way to get prepared is to make a list of your medical problems and the ways they have affected your life so that you'll be accurate, direct, and specific when talking to your doctor. Also, this way, you won't forget something you wanted to tell him (this can happen easily!). Of course, the allergist will have questions to ask you about your particular medical situation, but if you've thought about your problems in advance, it will foster clear communication between the two of you. It is as much your responsibility to be well prepared for your doctor appointment as it is your doctor's responsibility to listen to you and treat you with competence.

Consider these issues when you prepare what you'll tell your doctor about your health:

Breathing Problems Tell your doctor *what* your breathing problems have been, *how long* and *how often* you have had these problems, *how severe* the problems have been, *how* the problems have affected your life, and *if* and *when* you have had any symptom-free times. To help you clarify your breathing problems, think about these symptoms of asthma and use them as a guide:

- general shortness of breath;
- feelings of chest tightness;
- coughing (loose, tight, dry, or producing mucus);
- wheezing (which isn't always present with asthma); and
- nasal or throat problems (which are often associated with asthma).

It also helps if you consider whether your symptoms have been related to a cold or flu; exercise; exposure to irritating fumes; stress; weather changes; or potential allergens—such as animals, feathers, dust, pollen, and moulds.

Medicines You Are Taking If you are taking *any* medicines (over-the-counter or prescription) for *any* medical condition, tell your doctor about all of them. You need to tell the name of the medicine, the dosage strength, how often you take it, and what you're taking it for. (If you're taking antihistamines, stop taking them 24 hours before you see the allergist. Most likely, the allergist will administer skin tests to see if you have allergies, and antihistamines can interfere with skin-test readings.)

Questions about Your Condition Write down your specific concerns about your condition and don't hesitate to ask your allergist about them. Maybe some of your questions will be answered during your visit, but if some are not or if new questions arise as your visit progresses, bring them up to your allergist so that you can get the information you need to understand your condition.

What Will Happen During My Visit
to the Allergist?

When you visit an allergist, you can expect a thorough medical workup and evaluation, based upon your symptoms. The allergist will establish a diagnosis and then institute a long-range treatment program to meet your needs. For now, we'll look at how asthma is diagnosed. (We'll look at treatment measures in subsequent chapters.)

A diagnosis of asthma is based on your medical history, a careful and thorough physical exam, and laboratory tests.

MEDICAL HISTORY

An allergist finds out about your medical history by asking you questions about your present and past health problems, your family's medical history, your social and emotional history, and your environment. This is his way of learning about you, your immediate medical problems, and your past health conditions.

Present and Past Medical History A medical history is necessary for the doctor to learn about your symptoms (coughing, wheezing, and such), gain some measure of their severity, and determine whether they are consistent with a diagnosis of asthma. During this time, he will inquire about possible triggers for your asthma (suspected or unsuspected), and he will ask about other diseases or medicines that may or may not be affecting your asthma. By asking about your present illness patterns, he can gain an impression of the cause and severity of your asthma, and of other conditions that could be contributing to or causing your symptoms.

The allergist will want to know about any past hospitalizations or emergency room visits for asthma, and about any past medicines taken for asthma. He may ask if you've ever experienced any food intolerances, eczema, nasal problems, or sinus problems associated with your asthma. Additionally, he will ask if you've had any previous skin testing or allergy shots.

He will inquire about other illnesses or surgeries because they might affect the management of your asthma. Along the same line, he will ask about any drugs you are taking for other problems. Since a combination of certain drugs can have adverse effects, it's important for him to have this information before prescribing any medication for your asthma.

Family Medical History In Chapters 1 and 4, we discussed the importance of family history in terms of an allergic or asthmatic condition. If allergy or asthma runs in your family, you are likely to have them, too.

Your doctor will ask it there's a history of asthma or allergy in your family. If you inquire among the members of your family, you might be surprised to find how many of them had or have symptoms of allergy or asthma but never realized what they were.

Environmental History Knowing about your environment will help your allergist determine possible environmental triggers that could be provoking your asthma. He will ask you questions regarding your home and your work environments. He may even ask you questions about your hobbies. If it's your child who may have asthma, he may ask about his day-care facilities or his school. All of these kinds of questions are aimed at learning how and to what degree the environment contributes to the asthma symptoms. Here are some typical questions your doctor will ask, about:

- *dust triggers*
  - Do you have wall-to-wall carpeting? (Dust collects in carpet fibres and, when your carpet is vacuumed, gets stirred up into the air you breathe.)
  - Do you have an unusually dusty environment in your home?
- *mould triggers*
  - Do you have areas in your environment that facilitate mould growth? (Damp showers, basements, and uncovered crawl spaces, to mention a few.)
  - Do you have lots of house plants? (Their soil supports mould growth.)
  - Do you have fruit-storage areas in your environment? (Decaying and rotting fruit encourages mould growth.)
- *animal triggers*
  - Are you exposed to animals on a daily basis in your home, work, or school environments? (Indoor animals can be a major source of allergen, whereas outdoor animals usually don't cause much of a problem unless you are close to them.)
- *occupational or hobby-related triggers*
  - Do you work indoors or outdoors?
  - What indoor/outdoor hobbies do you enjoy?
  - In your job or hobbies, are you exposed to pollens, other allergic substances, or substances that might irritate your asthma?
- *other triggers*
  - Are you exposed to feather pillows or birds in your environment?
  - Are you exposed to stuffed furniture or jute-backed carpets in your environment? (Kapok used in furniture stuffing and jute fibres used as carpet backing are allergenic.)

Social and Emotional History As with any other chronic illness, asthma can have a considerable impact on your emotional responses and social interactions. Therefore, it's very important to discuss with your doctor your social and emotional history and the extent to which your asthma has affected it. Knowing this information helps your doctor treat you as a total person. These are some questions your doctor may ask you about this subject: How do you see your life changing when you have asthma? How do you cope with asthma? How do you feel about any limitations placed upon you and your life by asthma? In what ways do you change your life-style or activities when you're having problems with asthma? Are you experiencing any particular stress related to your home, school, or work life?

You need to be aware that your social and emotional well-being can affect your asthma. Social and emotional stress can worsen asthma. In a sense, this makes asthma psychosomatic (meaning that asthma's physical symptoms can result from stressful situations). More importantly, you need to be aware of the reverse: that asthma can affect your social and emotional well-being. In this respect, stress can result from having asthma. In a sense, this makes asthma somatopsychic (this means that stress symptoms can result from the physical illness of asthma).

Sometimes we don't think about the relationship between our social and emotional well-being and an illness. This relationship is very real. Thinking about it and talking about it openly to your doctor are steps in the direction of coping with your asthma and the stress that comes with it. (For more information about stress and asthma, refer to Chapter 15.)

PHYSICAL EXAMINATION

Your doctor will give you a thorough physical exam to discover further signs of asthma and other related conditions and to generally assess your physical health. Actually, much of a physical exam's findings simply confirm the information you gave in your history.

When looking for signs of asthma, your allergist will examine your:

- eyes
  - for dark circles beneath (sometimes seen in asthmatics and called "allergic shiners"), caused by nasal congestion, commonly associated with asthma;
  - for a wrinkle just beneath the lower eyelid, commonly called "Dennie's line" (often found in allergic asthmatics); and
  - for allergic conjunctivitis (an inflammation of the membranes around the eye).
- nose
  - for a crease above the tip of the nose, resulting from constantly rubbing it upwards with the palm of your hand to get relief from nasal itching (this is called the "allergic salute");

- for nasal blockage from polyps or membrane swelling;
- for signs of sinus problems with a device called a trans-illuminator, which is put into your mouth and illuminates your sinuses; and
- for other signs of nasal obstruction, such as a gaping facial expression that results from constant mouth breathing, or flared nostrils, as often seen with severe asthma symptoms.

- ears
  - for fluid behind the eardrum, which comes from nasal obstruction (this is common in asthmatics).
- mouth
  - for enlarged tonsils or adenoids (sometimes tonsils are enlarged in an asthmatic), which can cause noisy breathing and airflow obstruction and can contribute to infections.
- chest
  - for wheezing and sounds of mucus in the windpipes, while you blow out air in a forced, rapid way;
  - for a slight barrel-shaped chest (seen in chronic asthmatics), which comes from air trapping inside the lungs; and
  - for retraction of the breastbone and spaces between the ribs when breathing, which can occur with severe asthma symptoms.
- skin
  - for eczema (a common skin condition associated with allergy and asthma) on any part of your body, but especially found in the bends of your arms and knees.

Once he has completed your physical exam, your doctor will usually have an impression or a working diagnosis of your condition. He will then get laboratory tests to confirm his impressions.

Not only can lab tests confirm whether you have asthma, but they can determine how severe your asthma is, identify what many of your asthma triggers actually are, and uncover clues of other diseases that could be affecting your asthma.

LABORATORY TESTS FOR DIAGNOSING ALLERGY

The most common and simplest laboratory tests to diagnose allergy are *skin tests*. Skin tests are commonly given in the allergist's office and can quickly determine if you have allergies (common asthma triggers). These tests also help discover what allergens you should avoid in your environment and determine what allergens should be used in an allergy-shot treatment program, if later found to be necessary. Skin tests expose you to tiny amounts of potentially allergenic substances by applying them to your skin. If you're allergic to a substance, a reaction will occur in the form of a wheal (an itchy red and white swelling on your skin that resembles a mosquito bite).

Various techniques can be used for the skin tests. In a scratch test, allergens are applied to tiny scratches that penetrate only the very top layer of skin. These scratches don't hurt and don't bleed. They can be applied on your arms or back, can be read in 15 to 20 minutes, and form a wheal if positive. If a scratch test is negative, an intradermal skin test is used, which will pick up allergies missed by a scratch test. An intradermal skin test is done by injecting a tiny amount of allergen just under your skin. It causes little pain. An intradermal skin test can be read in 15 to 20 minutes and forms a wheal if positive, as with the scratch test.

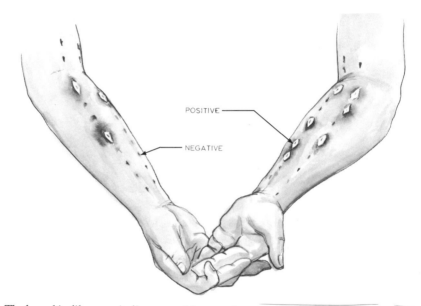

POSITIVE

NEGATIVE

The large hivelike areas indicate a positive reaction to a skin test, whereas the small dots signify a negative reaction.

Certain factors can affect skin testing:

Age Skin tests are less reactive in the under 3 age group and the elderly because people these ages often have less antibodies to the allergens tested.

Body rhythms Minor changes in skin-test reactions occur at different times of the day. Reactions are the least in the morning and the greatest in the evening.

Drugs Antihistamines can interfere with skin-test reactions; therefore, it's best to discontinue antihistamines 24 hours before having a skin test. (Antiasthma drugs and decongestants, on the other hand, don't significantly affect skin tests.)

Dermagraphic skin Skin that welts up easily from pressure alone can affect the accuracy of skin testing. Tell your doctor before skin tests are applied if you welt up easily after being scratched or from pressure on your skin, such as around your belt line.

Some allergists prefer doing a *RAST test* instead of skin tests. A RAST test (Radioallergosorbent test) is a sophisticated blood test that measures the small quantity of allergic antibody (IgE antibody) in the blood that will react with a specific allergen. One blood sample substitutes for numerous skin tests, but this is the RAST test's only advantage.

In terms of its disadvantages, RAST tests are less sensitive than skin tests and more expensive, and not enough individual RAST tests are available to test for all of the allergens in many areas. In addition, the results of RAST tests vary among different labs, and it generally takes too long to get results back. Even though the RAST can be an accurate and valuable tool in diagnosing allergy, we think skin tests are better.

You need to be aware of other methods used in attempts to diagnose allergies. Many of them have been used empirically for years, but have never met with any scientific verification that they truly diagnose allergy. We mention them here to caution you against them and for your general information on allergy testing.

Leukocytotoxic Testing This test consists of adding an allergen to an individual's blood sample that will result in a lowered white blood count if the person is allergic. Unfortunately, no reliability of the test has ever been demonstrated.

Subcutaneous Provocation Testing This consists of injecting into the arm suspected allergens in increasing doses until a person experiences symptoms. This is immediately followed by an injection, which is supposed to relieve these symptoms. Based on this information, allergy shots are prescribed for treatment. Several well-controlled studies have found these procedures to be of no help in diagnosing or treating allergy.

Sublingual Provocation Testing This test is based upon the same notion as the subcutaneous method, only the allergen is put under the person's tongue instead of injected. Advocates of this method claim it can be used for diagnosing and treating food allergies. Again, no well-controlled studies have found this procedure to be valid.

Rinkel Method This method involves skin testing by increasing the concentration of the test dose until a positive reaction can be read. Information from this testing is used to determine the starting dose and the optimal dose for allergy shots. Unfortunately, this method of testing leads to questionable diagnosis of allergy since the test result is often only an irritant reaction from the increasing strength of the testing material.

Also, starting and optimal allergy-shot doses predicted by this method result in doses too low to be effective in treating allergies.

The following laboratory tests *can* be used in an allergy evaluation, depending on your circumstances.

IgE Antibody Test This is a blood test that measures the total amount of the IgE antibody in the blood. High IgE levels can suggest allergy, but also other conditions, and low IgE levels don't necessarily rule out allergy. This test is basically used as a general screening by some physicians.

Eosinophil Count An eosinophil is a type of white blood cell that is often elevated in both kinds of asthma. However, it's elevated more in intrinsic (nonallergic) asthma than in extrinsic (allergic) asthma. Sometimes there is a relationship between an elevated count and the severity of asthma.

Nasal or Sputum Smear A smear of nasal discharge or sputum is placed on a glass slide and tested for eosinophils under a microscope. The smear is often positive in an asthmatic.

Immunoglobulin Test Occasionally the doctor may want to test for antibodies that fight infection (immunoglobulins). This is especially important with children who have a lot of sinus problems and bacterial pneumonias in addition to asthma symptoms since their immunoglobulins may be low.

Sweat Chloride Test This test diagnoses cystic fibrosis, which can present symptoms of wheezing that are similar to those of asthma. At first, asthma and cystic fibrosis might be confused; a sweat chloride test will rule cystic fibrosis in or out.

Alpha-1 Antitrypsin Test Alpha-1 antitrypsin is an enzyme that protects the lungs against the development of emphysema. Lack of this enzyme occasionally occurs in families and results in early emphysema—even in nonsmokers. People deficient in this enzyme often have asthma symptoms before the emphysema becomes apparent. This deficiency can be detected with a simple blood test.

Chest X-Ray While a chest X-ray can't diagnose asthma, it is useful in severe asthma to find complications and to help diagnose pneumonia. A routine chest X-ray is helpful to have as a baseline for future comparison, but chest X-rays don't need to be taken every time you have an asthma attack unless it's severe and lung complications of asthma are suspected. (Complications are discussed in Chapter 9.)

Sinus X-Ray A sinus X-ray is helpful when upper-respiratory tract infections aggravate asthma. Sinusitis is a common condition occurring with asthma, and can aggravate asthma symptoms. (Sinusitis without asthma can cause coughing attacks from post-nasal drip and can be confused with asthma.)

Pulmonary Function Tests Pulmonary function tests, which can be performed in your doctor's office, are used to diagnose asthma and measure the severity of an asthma attack. You perform this test by blowing air from your mouth into a tubelike apparatus connected to a machine called a spirometer. A spirometer measures the amount and speed of the air moving in and out of your lungs. A measurement of the maximum *amount* of air moved out of your lungs during exhalation is called the forced vital capacity (FVC). A measurement of the maximum *speed* of air moved out of your lungs during exhalation is called the forced expiratory volume (FEV,); it's the amount of air exhaled during the first second.

A simple pulmonary function test on an asthmatic usually shows a decrease in the speed and amount of air moving out of the lungs. An improvement of these measurements will occur after inhaling a drug that opens the bronchial tubes (a bronchodilator).

Asthma can't be diagnosed by a simple pulmonary function test if the asthmatic is symptom-free at the time of testing. When this happens, the doctor may do another kind of pulmonary function test, called a *bronchial provocation test*, which provokes the bronchial tubes into spasm if the person being tested is asthmatic. This is done by inhaling a chemical mist (made up of methacholine or histamine) or by performing exercise. After these maneuvers, an asthmatic will show a decrease in the speed and amount of air moving out of his lungs, whereas a nonasthmatic will not.

Peak Flowmeter In your home, you can monitor asthma by using a small instrument called a peak flowmeter, which measures the speed of air movement from the lungs. This instrument is inexpensive, and can be purchased through local medical supply outlets.

o   o   o

After visiting the allergist, you should have a sense of awareness and understanding about your condition. Once you've reached this understanding, you will be ready to arm yourself with treatment and control measures prescribed by your allergist. To supplement these measures, there are also many workable self-help methods you can use to control your asthma (see Chapters 8, 13, and 15).

6

Asthma, Bronchitis, and Emphysema—How To Tell the Difference

Helen is 57 years old. For 5 years now, she has experienced chronic nasal congestion, which usually has been diagnosed as a sinus infection. For the last year, she has also experienced a lot of coughing and shortness of breath. These symptoms have become more bothersome and an increasing source of concern for Helen. Her symptoms have been treated with antibiotics many times, but they didn't help. Whenever she gets a cold, her symptoms flare up. Sometimes, when she really feels bad, it's such an effort to breathe that she can't walk across a room.

Up until 6 months ago, she had been a two-packs-per-day cigarette smoker for all of her adult life. Smoking seemed to aggravate her symptoms, so she quit even though she found it very difficult. Lately, she had been wondering, could her symptoms possibly mean emphysema? If so, how severe was it? Could any other lung diseases be causing these symptoms? And another worry had plagued her—could her problem be treated?

With these symptoms and concerns in mind, she decided to see her doctor.

What Are the Most Common Lung Diseases and How Do They Differ?

Asthma, bronchitis, and emphysema are all common lung diseases that can give rise to the same symptoms Helen experienced—including wheezing, coughing, and shortness of breath. These symptoms are due to airway obstruction, which is the common denominator for all three diseases. But these diseases are all different; they have different causes, progressions, prognoses, and treatments.

Asthma is a *reversible* obstructive airway disease; bronchitis is a *partially reversible* obstructive airway disease; and emphysema is a *mostly irreversible* obstructive airway disease. However, since bronchitis and emphysema

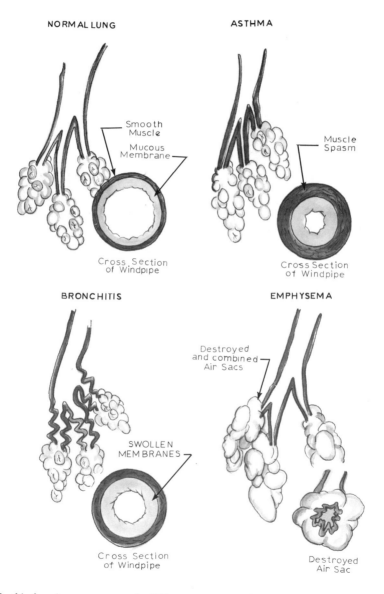

In this drawing, you can see the differences among asthma, bronchitis, and emphysema, and you can see how they compare to a normal state.

often have bronchospasm and increased mucous production, they often have an asthmatic component.

The development of airflow obstruction differs among asthma, bronchitis, and emphysema. In asthma, airflow obstruction results from contraction of the bronchial tubes, an increase in mucous production, and inflammation of the airways. These changes are reversible. With bronchitis, airflow obstruction results from inflammation of the airways with swelling of the mucous membranes and an increase in mucous production. These changes are often chronic and are only partially reversible. With emphysema, airflow obstruction is due to a breakdown of the air sacs, which results in their enlargement and subsequent loss of lung elasticity. Without their elasticity, the air sacs become limp and floppy and compress against the bronchioles (the smallest windpipes) making them collapse. These changes are mostly irreversible.

The prognosis is better for a person whose airflow obstruction is due to asthma or bronchitis than for one whose airflow obstruction is due to emphysema. With asthma, the response to treatment is generally good. With bronchitis, the response to treatment is not as good as with asthma, but much improvement in the condition can be achieved. Emphysema does not respond well to medication.

Bronchitis is frequently associated with some degree of emphysema because of their common major cause: cigarette smoking. If the individual stops smoking, his bronchitis may stop progressing and may even improve. Emphysema, on the other hand, will not improve when one stops smoking; however, its progression may slow down or come to a stop.

It's important to determine whether a person has asthma, bronchitis, or emphysema since proper diagnosis and subsequent treatment may make the difference between a normal, active life or a life with limitations.

How Does a Doctor Distinguish Among Asthma, Bronchitis, and Emphysema?

To distinguish among these airway-obstructive diseases, the doctor uses the patient's medical history, laboratory tests, and findings from his physical examination—paying special attention to the following areas:

Smoking History   The patient's smoking history is taken to determine his smoking habits and how they relate to the specific diseases. Asthmatics who smoke will notice a definite aggravation of symptoms when smoking, whereas those suffering from bronchitis and/or emphysema usually will not. Approximately three-fourths of the smokers who develop asthma will usually quit smoking on their own, and most of them will notice an improvement in symptoms soon after they stop. On the other hand, smokers who develop bronchitis and emphysema will notice little immediate improvement in their symptoms when they quit smoking, so they are usually less ready to quit on their own and almost always need outside encouragement.

Symptom Patterns Asthma's symptoms are of a paroxysmal nature (occurring in attacks or sudden recurrences), whereas the symptoms of bronchitis and emphysema are of a chronic nature (always present or with frequent recurrences).

Lab Tests and X-Rays Asthmatics will often have a high blood eosinophil count; a count over 400 usually signifies a reversible condition (asthma). Those with bronchitis and/or emphysema will not have an elevated eosinophil count. (Chest X-rays and other lab tests are usually of little value in distinguishing among these diseases.)

Pulmonary Function Tests These tests are used to directly determine the amount of reversibility of the obstructive airway disease. Usually the doctor will measure the forced vital capacity (lung volume) and the FEV_1 (amount of air that can be exhaled in 1 second), and then will administer a bronchodilator (an inhaled drug that opens the bronchial tubes). After the use of bronchodilators, asthmatics will usually experience a vast improvement in their pulmonary functioning. However, people with bronchitis will experience just a little improvement, and people with emphysema will not improve at all.

Physical Signs In addition to a patient's history and lab tests, certain findings from his physical exam can help the doctor distinguish among asthma, bronchitis, and emphysema. However, because of the frequency of overlap among these diseases, the physical findings often only give the doctor an impression of the disease causing the symptoms but no clear-cut diagnosis.

The doctor may not recognize the potential reversibility (indicating asthma) of the obstructive airway disease and may incorrectly diagnose the patient as having less reversible bronchitis or emphysema. Unfortunately, this results in an inaccurate poor prognosis, improper treatment, and a diminished quality of life for the patient, who, with the right diagnosis, could have been helped. The main value of distinguishing among asthma, bronchitis, and emphysema lies in establishing an accurate diagnosis with the right prognosis. This allows the doctor to prescribe the proper drug therapy to obtain the maximum reversibility of the obstructive airway disease.

In Summary, What Differences Exist Among Asthma, Bronchitis, and Emphysema?

The following are the general differences among asthma, bronchitis, and emphysema:

- Although asthma, bronchitis, and emphysema are all obstructive airway diseases, asthma is reversible, bronchitis is partially reversible, and emphysema is mostly irreversible.

- Their mechanisms of airflow obstruction differ. Bronchial hyperreactivity, contraction of bronchial tubes, and increased mucous production are responsible for airflow obstruction in asthma. Airway inflammation, swelling of mucous membranes, and increased mucous production are responsible for airflow obstruction in bronchitis. Loss of elasticity in the lungs and the collapse and destruction of tiny air sacs are responsible for airflow obstruction in emphysema.

- Smoking is without a doubt the major cause of bronchitis and emphysema, whereas it is only a trigger and source of aggravation for the asthmatic.

- The age of onset for asthma is usually younger than that for bronchitis and emphysema. However, asthma can start as late as age 70 or 80, and in certain cases bronchitis and emphysema can start as early as age 30.

- Their symptom patterns differ: Asthma symptoms are more paroxysmal, whereas symptoms for bronchitis and emphysema are more chronic.

- An elevated eosinophil count may indicate asthma; eosinophilia is not related to bronchitis or emphysema. The greater the eosinophil count, the greater the chance of obstructive airway reversibility.

- Nasal congestion with or without nasal polyps, sinusitis, and aspirin sensitivity are often associated with asthma; bronchitis and emphysema are usually partner to none of these conditions.

- Asthma responds well to drugs, bronchitis may respond somewhat to drugs, and emphysema does not respond to drugs.

- The prognosis is more optimistic for asthma and bronchitis since they are more treatable than emphysema. Emphysema cannot be reversed, so the prognosis, in this respect, is less optimistic; however, the general condition of a person with emphysema *can be improved*.

It is actually more helpful to determine the amount of the reversible component in the obstructive airway disease than to label the disease asthma, bronchitis, or emphysema. If *some* reversibility can be demonstrated, even if the major component of the disease is emphysema, then the proper medical treatment can be instituted to obtain maximum improvement. Undoubtedly, an accurate medical differentiation between the reversible and irreversible components of these obstructive airway diseases could make the difference between an individual being able to carry out the normal activities of daily living and work and his being disabled and dependent on others for help.

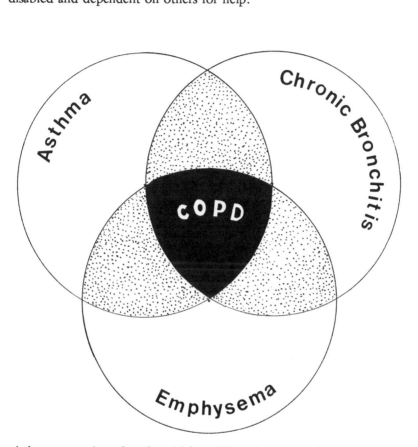

Asthma can coexist and overlap with bronchitis and emphysema because there are elements of bronchospasm and increased mucous production in all three diseases. Because they all cause obstruction to airflow, they are grouped under the name, chronic obstructive pulmonary disease, commonly referred to as COPD.

Caring for Asthma (in General and at Special Times)

7
Medications and Asthma

In this chapter, we'll take a good look at the medications that help an asthmatic lead a normal life. Medications are important "tools" in the treatment and control of asthma. As tools, they must be used properly to "fix" your asthma—you need to use the right medicines at the right times to achieve the best control of your asthma with minimal side effects.

When your doctor prescribes medications for your asthma, you need to know what the medications are and how to take them, how they work to help your asthma, and what possible side effects they carry with them.

You can use the information in this chapter to learn about and understand asthma medicines, answer questions you may have about the medicines, and calm any fears you may have about possible side effects. It's important for you to have this basic understanding so that you can use the medicine safely and effectively in treating and controlling your asthma.

What Are the Basic Asthma Medications?
Asthma medications fall into four basic categories:
- theophylline drugs (bronchodilators),
- beta-stimulator drugs (bronchodilators),
- cromolyn (antiallergic mediator agent), and
- steroids (anti-inflammatory agents).

Although there are four basic groups of drugs used to combat asthma, there are many drugs in each group and many different brand names for each drug. Don't let the myriad drug names confuse you. Once you understand the four basic categories explained in this chapter, you should have a good working knowledge about the way your asthma can be treated and managed with medications.

Remember, when asthma occurs, there is airway narrowing, airway inflammation, and large amounts of mucous production that plug the airways. Controlling asthma often involves the use of medicine to open the airways, decrease airway inflammation and mucous production, and encourage the clearing of mucus.

When To Take Asthma Medications

It's important to take medicine *as directed* by your doctor. If the prescription says to take it three times a day, take it as close to every 8 hours as possible, working it into your schedule (for instance, first thing in the morning, after school or work, and at bedtime).

If the prescription says to take it four times a day, take it as close to every 6 hours as possible, working it into your schedule. You might have to wake up during the night to take a needed dose if your asthma is severe. If your asthma is under control, you can work medicines around your sleep schedule (for instance, first thing in the morning, noon, dinnertime, and bedtime).

If the prescription says to take it two times a day, take it every 12 hours as best fits your schedule.

Long-acting asthma medications are usually taken one, two, or three time(s) a day, depending on the preparation used and how quickly your body metabolizes the drug. Short-acting asthma medications are usually taken every 4 to 6 hours.

Theophylline

Theophylline is a drug similar in some ways to caffeine, the substance in coffee and tea. It acts directly on the muscles of the airways to relax and open them. It does this by increasing an important chemical in the muscle cells of the airways. This chemical is called CAMP (cyclic adenosine 3'5' monophosphate). Its presence causes the airways to open and decreases the release of the harmful chemical mediators that cause asthma.

Theophylline has effects on other organs besides the lungs. For instance, it increases urine formation by the kidneys, increases acid in the stomach, relaxes the esophageal sphincter (the muscle that keeps the stomach contents out of the esophagus), increases the heart rate, and stimulates the nervous system. Usually these effects aren't noticeable, but on occasion can be bothersome.

WHAT IS THE USUAL DOSAGE OF THEOPHYLLINE?

The dose of theophylline depends on such factors as weight, age, presence of other diseases, and other medications being taken. Depending on these factors, the daily dose usually runs between 15 and 25 milligrams per kilogram of body weight (that's about 7 to 12 mg per pound of body weight), which is usually divided into several doses a day.

Theophylline is available in several forms. It comes in a liquid, in short-acting tablets, in long-acting tablets, and in a substance that can be sprinkled on food and swallowed. By a slight chemical modification, it can be changed to aminophylline, a form most commonly used intravenously. Also, it can be made into rectal suppositories, but this form isn't recommended because of its unpredictable absorption.

Certain factors alter the theophylline dosage requirement by increasing or decreasing the metabolism of the drug (the way the drug's broken down) by the liver. A person whose liver has a greater ability to metabolize theophylline will require a higher dose, and one whose liver is less able to metabolize the drug will require a lower dose.

The following factors require a higher theophylline dose because they cause the liver to metabolize the drug faster:

- younger age (except infants under 6 months),
- cigarette and marijuana smoking,
- concomitant use of other drugs, such as phenobarbital (Luminal) and phenytoin (Dilantin), and
- high protein diets.

These factors, on the other hand, require a lower theophylline dose because they cause the liver to metabolize the drug slower:

- viral illnesses or viral vaccinations (flu shots),
- fever,
- congestive heart failure,
- liver disease,
- older age and infants under 6 months,
- high-carbohydrate diet, and
- concomitant use of other drugs (including erythromycin [E-Mycin, EES, Ilosone, and Erythrocin], troleandomycin [Tao], ciprofluxacin [Cipro], cimetidine [Tagamet], and allopurinol [Zyloprim], as well as beta-blocking drugs such as metoprolol [Lopressor] and propranolol [Inderal]).

HOW LONG DOES IT TAKE FOR THEOPHYLLINE TO START WORKING?

Other than intravenously, the fastest absorption of theophylline occurs with the liquid forms, which reach their maximum effect in about 30 to 60 minutes. Maximum effect for short-acting tablets takes about 60 to

120 minutes; maximum effect for long-acting tablets takes anywhere from 4 to 16 hours, depending on the preparation used.

WHAT ARE THE SIDE EFFECTS OF THEOPHYLLINE?

Side effects are undesirable effects that may occur when usual and standard doses of a medicine are taken.

Some usual side effects of theophylline are:

- gastrointestinal (mild nausea, and heartburn),
- nervous system (headaches, restlessness, insomnia, muscle spasms, anxiety, irritability, and tremulousness),
- cardiovascular (rapid heartbeat [palpitations]), and
- others (excess perspiration and frequent urination).

These side effects usually go away as your body adjusts to the medicine. However, check with your doctor if any of them become particularly bothersome or persistent.

Toxic side effects occur when a medicine's dose is too high and the blood level gets above the desired therapeutic level (10 to 20 micrograms per millilitre of blood). Toxic side effects are exaggerated and more dramatic forms of the usual side effects just listed. Toxic side effects are severe, are not tolerated well, and our bodies do not adjust to them as they do with the usual side effects.

If you suspect toxic side effects, stop taking the medicine immediately and consult your doctor about a dosage adjustment.

WHAT YOUR DOCTOR SHOULD KNOW BEFORE YOU TAKE THEOPHYLLINE

Tell your doctor if you have any form of:

- liver or heart disease (this will require a lower dose of theophylline),
- gastritis or ulcer disease (theophylline increases acid secretion in the stomach), or
- esophagitis and/or hiatal hernia (theophylline increases acid secretion in the stomach and relaxes the sphincter between the stomach and esophagus, allowing acid to back up into the esophagus and cause heartburn).

Tell your doctor if you are taking these medicines:

- phenobarbital (Luminal) or
- phenytoin (Dilantin).

These drugs may require a higher dose of theophylline because they increase the metabolism of theophylline in the liver.

Tell your doctor if you are taking:

- erythromycin (E-Mycin, EES, Erythrocin, or Ilosone),

- troleandomycin (Tao capsules),
- ciprofluxacin (Cipro),
- cimetidine (Tagamet),
- allopurinol (Zyloprim), or
- beta-blocking drugs.

These drugs may require a lower dose of theophylline because they decrease the metabolism of theophylline in the liver.

Also, tell your doctor if you are taking:
- lithium (Eskalith or Lithane),
- beta-blocking drugs, or
- phenytoin (Dilantin).

The effects of these drugs are decreased by theophylline.

USE OF THEOPHYLLINE DURING PREGNANCY

Safety using theophylline during pregnancy hasn't definitely been established, but no known adverse effects in humans have ever been demonstrated. With asthma, the benefits of this drug outweigh the risks. However, it's best to tell your doctor if you are pregnant.

USE OF THEOPHYLLINE WHILE NURSING

Theophylline is present in mother's milk, but at lower concentrations than in plasma. It is safe to nurse, but it's best to nurse just before taking theophylline, since this is the time when the level in the milk would be lowest.

HABIT-FORMING POTENTIAL OF THEOPHYLLINE

None.

EFFECTS OF FOOD, BEVERAGES, AND TOBACCO ON THEOPHYLLINE

Food A high-protein diet increases the metabolism of theophylline and may result in the need for a higher dose, whereas a high-carbohydrate diet decreases the metabolism of theophylline and may result in the need for a lower dose. Avoid large amounts of chocolate, which contains caffeine. Caffeine may add to the adverse nervous system side effects of theophylline.

Nonalcoholic beverages Avoid large intakes of caffeine-containing beverages—such as tea, coffee, and cola drinks—when taking theophylline.

Alcoholic beverages None.

Tobacco Smoking increases the metabolism of theophylline, usually resulting in the need for a higher dose.

WHAT DRUGS ARE COMMONLY USED AS THEOPHYLLINE PREPARATIONS?

The following is a comprehensive list of commonly used theophylline preparations available to patients upon a doctor's prescription. The drugs are separated based on the percentage of their pure theophylline content, and listed by generic and brand names. Basically, there is no significant advantage of one over the other. However, aminophylline is easier to give intravenously because it is the most water-soluble.

The theophylline content of the drug preparation is taken into consideration when a dosage of the drug is calculated. Dosage is always based on the pure theophylline preparation, and adjustments in dosage are made appropriately depending on which theophylline preparation is used. For instance, a dose of oxtriphylline would be about a third higher than a dose of pure theophylline.

Theophylline

Generic name	Brand name	Content %
theophylline	Immediate-release preparations:	100%
	Aquaphyllin	
	Somophyllin-T	
	Bronkodyl	
	Elixophyllin	
	Theophyl	
	Slo-Phyllin (plain)	
	Theoclear 80 syrup	
	Theostat	
	Quibron-T	
	Accubron	
	Marax*	
	Tedral*	
	Aerolate (liquid)	
	Time-release preparations:	
	Aerolate (capsules)	
	Bronkodyl S-R	
	Constant-T	
	Elixophyllin SR	
	La BID	
	Quibron-T/SR	
	Respbid	
	Slo-bid Gyrocaps	
	Slo-Phyllin Gyrocaps	
	Somophyllin-CRT	
	Theobid Duracaps	
	Theoclear L.A. Capsules	

Generic name	Brand name	Content %
	Theo-Dur	
	Theolair-SR	
	Theospan-SR	
	Theovent	
	Theo-24	
	Uniphyl	
theophylline calcium salicylate	Quadrinal* Verequad*	48%
theophylline sodium glycinate	Asbron Synophylate	50%
oxtriphylline	Immediate-release preparations: Choledyl Brondecon* Time-release preparation: Choledyl SA	65%
dyphylline	Immediate-release preparations: Lufyllin Dilor Neothylline Droxine Time-release preparation: Droxine L.A.	Action is like theophylline, but dyphylline isn't a theophylline.
theophylline ethylenediamine	Immediate-release preparations: Somophyllin liquid Amesec* Time-release preparations: Aminodur Dura-Tabs Phyllocontin	80–85%

*These medications are combination drugs, consisting of a theophylline preparation combined with other medication.

Beta Stimulators

Beta stimulators have been around since the time of the ancient Chinese, when they used the herb *ma-huang*, whose major active chemical was later found to be ephedrine, a popular drug used for the treatment of asthma for many years. Although not a pure beta stimulator, ephedrine was the first drug of this class that could be used by mouth in the treatment of asthma.

Beta stimulators are very effective bronchodilators, and are a class of drugs often referred to as *sympathomimetic bronchodilators* because they have an adrenalinelike effect and work through the sympathetic nervous system.

With asthma, our bronchial tubes are tight and constricted. During an attack, our body's own adrenal output increases in response to the asthma attack. This stimulates the sympathetic nervous system, which causes the relaxation of the bronchial tubes and opens the airways. As with adrenaline, beta stimulators stimulate the sympathetic nervous system (hence, the term sympathomimetic) and cause the windpipes to relax. Also, beta stimulators inhibit the release of harmful chemical mediators that cause asthma.

Beta stimulators affect other organ systems in the body. For instance, they increase the rate and force of contraction of the heart, and relax the intestinal track and uterus.

HOW AND IN WHAT DOSAGE ARE BETA STIMULATORS TAKEN?

These drugs are taken by inhalation and injection and orally. The choice of preparation and means of administration will vary according to the asthmatic's needs. In general, the inhaled and injected preparations have a more rapid onset of action and a shorter duration of action than the oral forms, and are more helpful for acute asthma. The following tables list available drugs that are in part or whole beta stimulators.

Solutions for Machine-Driven Nebulization (Motorized Nebulizer) for Inhalation

Generic name	Brand name	Dosage
isoproterenol solution (isoprenaline)	Isuprel	.25 ml in 3 ml of salt water
metaproterenol solution (orciprenaline)	Alupent	.2–.3 ml in 3 ml of salt water
isoetharine solution	Bronkosol	.25–.5 ml in 3 ml of salt water
albuterol solution (salbutamol)	Ventolin, Proventil	.25–.5 ml in 3 ml of salt water

Note: Solutions given by a machine-driven nebulizer are usually helpful in an acute attack to obtain quicker and more complete penetration of the drugs than can be obtained with hand-held inhalers.

Inhaled Beta Stimulators

These have a quicker onset of action with generally less side effects than those given by mouth. Inhaled bronchodilators are usually used on an "as needed" basis.

Generic name	Brand name	Contents	Recommended dose	Onset of action (minutes)	Peak action (minutes)	Duration of action (hours)
epinephrine (adrenaline)	Medihaler-Epi Primetine, Bronkaid	0.3 mg/puff 0.2 mg/puff .25 mg/puff	1–2 puffs every 4 hrs. 1–2 puffs every 4 hrs. 1–2 puffs every 4 hrs.	2 mins.	5 mins.	1–2 hrs.
isoproterenol (isoprenaline)	Isuprel	0.125 mg/puff	1–2 puffs up to 5 times per day	2 mins.	5–30 mins.	
	Medihaler-Iso	0.075 mg/puff	1–2 puffs 4–6 times per day			
metaproterenol (orciprenaline)	Alupent, Metaprel	0.65 mg/puff	1–2 puffs every 4–6 hrs.	5 mins.	30–90 mins.	1–5 hrs.
isoetharine	Bronkometer	0.34 mg/puff	1–2 puffs every 4 hrs.	5 mins.	15–60 mins.	1–3 hrs.
albuterol, (salbutamol)	Ventolin, Proventil	0.09 mg/puff	1–2 puffs every 6–8 hrs.	5 mins.	30–60 mins.	4–6 hrs.
terbutaline	Brethaire	0.2 mg/puff	2 puffs every 4–6 hrs.	5 mins.	60–120 mins.	3–4 hrs.
bitolterol	Tornalate	0.37 mg/puff	2 puffs every 6–8 hrs.	3–4 mins.	30–60 mins.	6–7 hrs.

Note: Overuse of *any* of these inhalers may be dangerous.

Oral Beta Stimulators

It takes longer for oral beta stimulators to work since they must be absorbed first.

Generic name	Brand name	Content	Recommended dose	Onset of action	Peak of action	Duration of action
ephedrine	Many available	Varies according to preparation	15–50 mg 4–6 times/ day	30 mins.	2–3 hrs.	4–6 hrs.
metaproterenol (orciprenaline)	Alupent, Metaprel	10, 20 mg (Liquid: 10 mg/ tsp)	10–20 mg every 6–8 hours	30 mins.	2–2.5 hrs.	4–6 hrs.
terbutaline	Brethine, Bricanyl	2.5, 5 mg	2.5–5 mg every 6–8 hours	30 mins.	2–3 hrs.	4–6 hrs.
albuterol (salbutamol)	Ventolin, Proventil	2, 4 mg (Liquid: 2 mg/ tsp)	2–4 mg every 6–8 hours	30 mins.	1–3 hrs.	4–6 hrs.

Injectable Beta Stimulators

These are only used in acute situations, usually on a one-time basis to reverse an asthma attack.

Generic name	Brand name	Recommended dose	Onset of action	Peak action	Duration of action
epinephrine (adrenaline)	Adrenalin (various preparations)	0.2–.3 ml SC*	5 min.	1 hr.	1–4 hrs.
	Sus-Phrine	0.05–.3 ml SC*	10–15 min.	2 hrs.	8–10 hrs.
terbutaline	Bricanyl, Brethine	0.25 mg SC*	5–15 min.	0.5–1 hr.	1.5–4 hrs.

*SC means subcutaneously (beneath the skin).

WHAT ARE THE SIDE EFFECTS OF BETA STIMULATORS?

Some common side effects may occur with beta stimulators that usually do not require medical attention. These side effects may go away during treatment as your body adjusts to the medication. Beta stimulators have no long-term side effects, but you should check with your doctor if any side effects continue or become particularly bothersome.

Common side effects are:

- nervousness,
- headache,
- trembling,
- fast and pounding heart,
- dizziness or light-headedness,
- dryness or irritation of the mouth and throat,
- heartburn, and
- bad taste in mouth.

Toxic side effects of beta stimulators are exaggerations of the common side effects just listed.

WHAT YOUR DOCTOR SHOULD KNOW BEFORE YOU TAKE BETA STIMULATORS

Inform your doctor if you have any form of:

- heart disease (beta stimulators may aggravate irregular heart rhythms or angina pectoris [chest pain of heart disease]),
- hyperthyroidism or hypertension (beta stimulators may aggravate both of these conditions), or
- diabetes (beta stimulators may increase blood sugar minimally, but generally should cause no concern).

Inform your physician if you are taking other medications. For instance, beta stimulators may cause active seizures or a hypertensive crisis in people on MAO inhibitors (Parnate, Marplan, and Nardil).

USE OF BETA STIMULATORS DURING PREGNANCY

Safety hasn't definitely been established with the use of beta stimulators during pregnancy. However, no known adverse effects in humans have ever been demonstrated, with exception of a very rare association of epinephrine with congenital abnormalities if used during the first 4 months of pregnancy. With asthma, the benefits of these drugs usually outweigh the risks, but it's best to tell your doctor if you are pregnant.

Inhaled beta stimulators are theoretically safer than oral forms because they have less of a systemic effect. In late pregnancy, the use of beta stimulators has the potential for delaying the onset of labor, but this hasn't proven to be a problem with the usual dosage used in asthma treatment.

USE OF BETA STIMULATORS WHILE NURSING

It's unknown whether these drugs are present in human milk. No known adverse reactions have been demonstrated in humans, but it's best to consult your doctor if you are nursing.

HABIT FORMING POTENTIAL OF BETA STIMULATORS

None.

EFFECTS OF FOOD, BEVERAGES, AND TOBACCO ON BETA STIMULATORS

Food None.

Nonalcoholic beverages Avoid large intakes of caffeine-containing beverages, such as tea, coffee, and cola drinks. They may add to the adverse nervous system side effects of beta stimulators.

Alcoholic beverages None.

Tobacco None.

WHAT DRUGS ARE COMMONLY USED AS BETA-STIMULATOR PREPARATIONS?

Refer to the tables on pages 83–86.

Cromolyn

Cromolyn is a unique antiasthmatic and antiallergic drug. Cromolyn is derived from khellin, a natural drug extracted from *Ammi visnaga*, an Eastern Mediterranean herb. It has been used in Europe since the 1960s and in the United States since 1970. Cromolyn is known by the brand name Intal and is a useful agent in treating some asthmatics.

Cromolyn acts by preventing mediator release from mast cells that have been triggered by an allergic reaction. It also prevents some nonallergic-triggered mediator release, such as that which occurs with exercise-induced asthma. To be effective, it must be used before there is contact with the triggering stimulus. Along with preventing mediator release, it seems to reduce bronchial hyperreactivity.

It is used mostly to treat extrinsic (allergic) asthma, but it also works well on some nonallergic triggers for asthma, such as exercise, and it may be of some benefit to the intrinsic (nonallergic) asthmatic.

WHAT IS THE USUAL DOSAGE OF CROMOLYN?

The usual dosage for cromolyn is 20 milligrams four times per day, administered as a powdered aerosol diluted in lactose (milk sugar). It's inhaled through an apparatus, called a *Spinhaler*, that propels the powder into the lungs as it is inhaled deeply and rapidly. Cromolyn can also be administered by a hand-held inhaler at a dose of 1.6 milligrams (two puffs) four times per day, which gives the same effect as 20 milligrams from Spinhaler. For small children, it can be given by nebulization of a solution with a motorized nebulizer at a dose of 20 mg four times per day.

WHAT ARE THE SIDE EFFECTS OF CROMOLYN?

Cromolyn is relatively free of all short- and long-term side effects, with a few exceptions: Its powdery substance may produce minor throat irritation and may trigger mild asthma symptoms. However, the latter side effect can usually be prevented by inhaling a beta stimulator prior to inhaling cromolyn.

WHAT YOUR DOCTOR SHOULD KNOW BEFORE YOU TAKE CROMOLYN

There are no adverse interactions between cromolyn and other drugs. However, tell your doctor if you have a liver or kidney disease because the dose may need to be lowered.

USE OF CROMOLYN DURING PREGNANCY

No adverse effects on pregnancy have ever been demonstrated. The benefits of this medicine during pregnancy outweigh the risks.

USE OF CROMOLYN WHILE NURSING

It's not known if cromolyn is present in human milk. No adverse reactions have been reported with the use of this drug in lactating women. The benefits of cromolyn usually outweigh the risks.

HABIT FORMING POTENTIAL OF CROMOLYN

None.

EFFECTS OF FOOD, BEVERAGES, AND TOBACCO ON CROMOLYN

Food None.

Nonalcoholic beverages None.

Alcoholic beverages None.

Tobacco None.

WHAT DRUGS ARE COMMONLY USED AS CROMOLYN PREPARATIONS?

Intal in 20-mg capsules, Intal used in a hand-held inhaler, and Intal in 20-

mg ampules for use in a motorized nebulizer are common cromolyn preparations.

Steroids

Steroids include a large group of hormones made in our bodies by the ovaries, testicles, and the adrenal glands. Steroids have an effect on many of our body's functions. There are three large groups of steroid hormones, which differ from each other in both their medical effects and side effects:

Estrogen and progestins   These steroid hormones are produced in the ovary and the adrenal gland, and function as female hormones.

Androgenic (anabolic) steroids, such as testosterone   Produced mainly by the testicle, but also by the ovary and adrenal gland, these steroids function as male hormones. Athletes have taken anabolic steroids when they've tried to improve their physical prowess with drugs.

Adrenocorticosteroids   These steroids are produced by the adrenal gland only. They influence many of our organs and tissues to rapidly adapt to our constantly changing environment and therefore allow our bodies to perform with relative freedom. Without adrenocorticosteroids, our bodies could function only under very rigid conditions; for example, we would need to consume exact amounts of salt daily, eat food in small amounts at all times, and maintain environmental temperatures within a very narrow range.

When we speak of steroids in this section, we will only be referring to adrenocorticosteroids.

Steroids are produced normally in our body by the adrenal glands every day. In times of stress or during times of illness, our normal body response is to increase the production of steroids to compensate for the unusual imbalance placed on our bodies. By means of technical advances over the last 40 years, the pharmaceutical industry has been able to synthesize chemicals that are the same or have similar actions as our natural steroid, cortisol. One of these chemicals is the commonly used steroid, *prednisone*. The amount of natural steroid (cortisol) our bodies produce every day is equal to about 7.5 milligrams of prednisone.

Steroid drugs are powerful agents with the potential for causing great benefit as well as great harm. Since their introduction, they have probably been used for a greater range of maladies than any other class of drug. When steroid drugs were first being used, there was a lack of carefully controlled clinical trials to assess their risks and benefits. Not surprisingly, this left doctors little information on the appropriate and rational use of steroid drugs. But gradually over the years, the necessary scientific knowledge for determining a more rational therapy with steroids has become available so that doctors can now employ and administer them in a safer manner. This is especially true as regards the use of steroids in the treatment of asthma.

HOW DO STEROIDS ACT IN THE BODY?

Steroids make cells perform a function that they ordinarily couldn't do alone. They do this through a very complex mechanism by attaching themselves to a cell's DNA (deoxyribonucleic acid) and thereby altering the cell's function. These alterations result in many different actions throughout the body. For our purposes, we'll only discuss the actions that are beneficial for asthmatics. In asthmatics, steroids:

- increase the action of beta-stimulating drugs and natural beta-stimulating chemicals in the body to dilate the windpipes,
- decrease the inflammation in and around the windpipes, and
- retard the formation of chemical mediators that cause inflammation and bronchospasms.

WHAT IS THE USUAL DOSAGE OF STEROIDS?

The steroid most often used to treat asthma is prednisone. The dosage depends on the severity and duration of the asthma attack.

For Severe Asthma Attacks   The dosage requirement may be as much as 6 to 12 milligrams per kilogram of body weight per day (that is about 3 to 6 mg per pound of a person's body weight). Further dosages depend on the person's response to the treatment. For instance, if your asthma clears up quickly, the dosage can be tapered to lower doses. If you don't get better, you may need higher doses for several days until you improve.

For Moderate Asthma Attacks   For adults, the starting dosage is 40 to 80 milligrams per day. This dosage is continued for 2 to 3 days, and then tapered over the next 10 days to a dose of 10 mg per day or less, or 30 mg every other day or less, or stopped completely. The starting dosage for children is .5 to 1 milligram per kilogram of body weight per day, and then it's tapered in a similar way.

For Chronic Asthma   Sometimes a maintenance dose of prednisone is required for months or years to keep asthma symptoms under reasonable control. Under these circumstances, it's best to use the lowest dose possible that still controls asthma, and if possible, to use it on an alternate-day schedule. Chronic asthma can usually be controlled on a dose of less than 10 milligrams per day or less than 30 milligrams every other day. The best maintenance dosage usually must be worked out by trial and error.

HOW LONG DOES IT TAKE FOR STEROIDS TO WORK?

Prednisone can give some beneficial effects within 12 hours. However, sometimes it may take as long as 2 weeks before you'll notice a significant effect.

WHAT ARE SOME COMMONLY USED STEROID PREPARATIONS?

See the table on page 94.

WHAT ARE THE SIDE EFFECTS OF STEROIDS?

People often worry about the possible side effects of steroids in treating asthma. However, systemic side effects of steroids are mostly the result of long-term high-dose use. The short-course treatment—so often essential in controlling a severe attack of asthma or in preventing a moderate attack from evolving into a severe life-threatening one—rarely, if ever, causes significant side effects.

There are no toxic doses for steroids. Obviously, when very high doses must be used over long periods of time, more frequent and severe side effects will occur. But since asthma, for the most part, doesn't usually require the high doses other diseases may necessitate, the possible side effects are much less frequent and severe. Nonetheless, you need to recognize and understand the side effects of steroids, should they occur.

The following list of steroids' side effects is long, but complete. We include all of the possible side effects to give you a full picture of them and their relationship to the usual treatment doses used in controlling asthma.

Personality Changes These changes vary in degree from insomnia, nervousness, and slight mood changes to severe manic and/or depressive reactions. However, these side effects are more likely to occur in someone with tendencies towards these problems. Severe personality changes are rare, and mild personality changes usually subside even when steroids are continued. At any rate, these side effects generally go away when steroids are stopped. Low daily doses or alternate-day doses infrequently cause these personality problems.

Nervous System Side Effects Symptoms of headache, nausea, vomiting, and blurred vision can occur from a rare complication associated with steroid use, known as pseudotumor cerebri, which is an increased pressure in the cavities of the brain. This rare condition generally occurs *after* steroids are stopped rapidly. It is corrected by reinstituting steroids and then starting a slower tapering dose.

Side Effects of the Eye There's an increased incidence of cataracts, especially with prolonged use (more than one year) of high-dose steroids; this incidence is approximately 6 percent. The incidence of cataracts is uncommon with less than 10 milligrams per day or with an alternate-day treatment schedule.

For some reason, asthmatics who use steroids are less likely to develop cataracts than people who use comparable doses of steroids for other medical conditions.

While steroids can cause cataracts, this is not the worst of all possible side effects, because they usually do not continue to form after steroids are stopped and they may even go away. Should you need high-dose long-term steroids and cataracts occur, consult an ophthalmologist. Cataract surgery is a viable option.

In some people, steroids can raise the pressure in the eye, which can result in glaucoma. However, this occurs only when using topical steroids applied directly to the eyes, and reverses when they're withdrawn. Glaucoma does not occur with steroids taken by mouth or injection when used for asthma.

Gastrointestinal Side Effects   Contrary to popular belief, steroids don't commonly produce ulcer disease. Some studies show no relationship between steroids and ulcer disease, whereas others suggest a slight increase in ulcer disease with steroids. At the very worst, high steroid doses can be rare inducers of peptic ulcer disease.

On the other hand, steroids can cause minor gastric irritation. And steroids have been implicated as a cause of pancreatitis (inflammation of the pancreas), but the prospect of this is rare.

Metabolic and Endocrine Side Effects

Increased appetite and weight gain   Steroids cause increased appetite and weight gain in many people. The higher the dose, the greater the appetite stimulation. Even with low daily or alternate-day doses, some people gain weight while taking steroids.

Effects on blood glucose   Steroids can cause elevation of blood sugar by increasing the production of glucose by the liver and by decreasing the metabolism (breakdown) of glucose by the body tissue. This steroid-induced elevation of blood glucose is not the same as true diabetes, and has none of the ramifications of true diabetes other than the elevated blood sugar, and is completely reversible after the dose is lessened or stopped. With the use of alternate-day low-dose steroids, the effects on elevated blood glucose are usually mild unless you are a diabetic.

Effects on fat distribution   Large doses of steroids can cause a peculiar alteration in fat distribution, commonly referred to as a *cushingoid state*. With this state, there may be a gain of fat deposits in the back of the neck, known as a "buffalo hump"; in the cheeks, resulting in a "moon face"; and in areas just above the collarbone. In contrast to all of this, there may also

Commonly Used Steroid Preparations

Generic name	Brand name	Duration	Relative Potency*
prednisone	Deltasone	short-acting (24 hrs.)	5 mg
	Liquid Pred Syrup		
prednisolone	Pediapred (liquid)	short-acting (24 hrs.)	5 mg
	Prelone Syrup	short-acting (24 hrs.)	5 mg
	Roxane		
methylprednisolone	Medrol	short-acting (24 hrs.)	4 mg
hydrocortisone		short-acting (24 hrs.)	20 mg
triamcinolone	Aristocort	long-acting (36 hrs.)	4 mg
dexamethasone	Decadron	long-acting (45 hrs.)	.75 mg
	Dexasone		
	Hexadroal		
betamethasone	Celestone	long-acting (45 hrs.)	.6 mg

*Relative potency of steroid preparations are based on 5 mg of prednisone.

be a loss of fat from the extremities. Usually these effects are mild, and rarely occur when using alternate-day or low daily doses in controlling asthma. If these side effects do occur, they would be completely reversible when the steroids are stopped.

On occasion, steroids can cause increased blood triglycerides to a moderate degree and blood cholesterol to a mild degree, but no known heart disease has been associated with steroids.

Water and electrolyte changes Prolonged or high doses of steroids cause salt retention by the kidneys. As a consequence, water is retained to balance the sodium retention and this may result in some mild swelling of the feet, hands, and face. In large doses, steroids can cause potassium loss by the kidney.

Menstrual irregularities Menstrual irregularities occasionally can occur with the use of steroids. This is usually with high doses or prolonged use. You should make certain to rule out other causes for menstrual irregularities before assuming they are due to steroids.

Adrenal suppression Remember that steroids are made by our adrenal glands at equivalent doses of 7.5 milligrams of prednisone per day. Doses equal to or in excess of this amount on a daily basis may suppress the body's own adrenal glands from producing steroids. This could be dangerous because an increase of steroids from the adrenal gland is necessary to help our bodies cope in times of trauma, stress, or infection. Suppression of the adrenal gland's production of steroids can be avoided by using a single dose of steroids every other day in the morning or a low daily dose of 7.5 milligrams (or less) of prednisone.

When your doctor prescribes alternate-day steroids, make sure they are short-acting steroids, such as prednisone, because long-acting steroids will cause adrenal suppression even if given on an alternate-day basis. These are some common short-acting steroids:

- prednisone (Deltasone and Orasone),
- prednisolone (Delta-Cortef and Sterane),
- methylprednisolone (Medrol), and
- hydrocortisone.

If you are taking steroids for extended periods of time, especially in a dose range that will suppress your adrenal gland function, most doctors will give you higher doses during times of trauma, stress, or infection.

Growth suppression Steroids may suppress growth if taken on a daily basis at a high enough dose to suppress the adrenal gland. When taken on alternate days, there is little growth suppression. Remember that asthma, per se, also suppresses growth; therefore, sometimes it is difficult to determine which is most responsible for growth suppression. Actually, it's not uncommon to see a spurt of growth with the use of steroids as the asthma comes under control. Parents needn't be concerned about growth suppression when low-dose daily steroids (less than 7.5 milligrams) or alternate-day steroids (at any dose) are used.

Skin Problems

Acne   Steroids can produce an acnelike rash, found mostly over the shoulders, chest, and back. This is more common with adolescents who are acne prone. Acne problems clear up after steroids are stopped. Acne is usually not a significant problem with low or alternate-day doses.

Hirsutism   Steroids can cause hair growth in unusual places, such as the face and back, in those who are genetically more likely to grow hair. This usually isn't a problem with low or alternate-day doses.

Thinning of skin   Steroids can result in skin thinning, especially in the elderly, with long-term use (longer than 3 months).

Bruising of skin   Increased bruising can result from fragile capillaries in the skin that break more easily on contact. This is common in the elderly with fair-complected skin. Increased bruising can occur with the lower doses used in asthma treatment.

Impaired wound healing   Wound healing can be impaired with *large doses* of steroids if taken longer than 3 months, but low daily or alternate-day doses have little effect on wound healing.

Striae   Sometimes people on long-term high-dose steroids can develop bluish purple lines over their flanks and thighs, known as striae. After steroids are stopped, they become less noticeable, but don't completely go away. Striae can also occur normally, especially in obese individuals, and in association with other diseases.

Sweating   Increased sweating may be an irritation for you if you're taking steroids.

Musculoskeletal Side Effects

Osteoporosis   Steroids may cause a reduction in bone mass, which is known as osteoporosis. The incidence of problems with osteoporosis—such as collapse of a vertebrae with back pain or bone fractures—is low (less than 4 percent) when doses of 10 milligrams (or less) of prednisone per day are used for up to 5 years, whereas its incidence is much higher (up to 40 percent) when high doses of 30 milligrams (or more) per day are used for more than one year.

Although steroids can decrease bone mass, this is usually minimal with the lower doses used to treat asthma. There's a greater risk of osteoporosis developing in association with the use of steroids in the elderly, in those with diseases that cause immobility, and in postmenopausal women because their bone mass is marginal to begin with. Vitamin D and calcium supplements may prevent problems of osteoporosis, and should be used by those in these higher risk groups. Estrogen may also be a preventive measure, but check with your doctor for this information.

Two easily performed procedures for detection of early osteoporosis have recently been made readily available. One is the photon densitometer and the other is a modified CAT scan of the spine. Both of these noninvasive, painless procedures are effective in detecting early bone loss.

Aseptic bone necrosis This condition is a necrosis (death of living tissue) of part of the hipbone, caused from a decrease in blood supply to the hipbone. It is seen commonly in alcoholics and in those who suffer hip fractures. In addition, it is seen in association with many other conditions, such as lupus erythematosus, rheumatoid arthritis, sickle cell anemia, hemophilia, polycythemia, radiation injury, gout, diabetes, and renal transplants.

It is reported to be a rare complication of steroids when used at high doses for a long duration. In most cases it is difficult to determine whether an underlying condition or the steroids themselves caused the aseptic necrosis. It is rare to find this condition in an asthmatic taking steroids who doesn't have any other complicating conditions that could also be causing the aseptic necrosis.

Myopathy This is a weakness of the muscles, especially of the upper legs. It occurs more commonly as a complication of the drug triamcinolone, which is a longer acting steroid than the more commonly used prednisone. This condition is usually associated with high doses of steroids, and may improve after they are tapered off or stopped.

Cardiovascular Complications Steroids have no direct effects on the heart, but because they cause sodium retention, they can increase fluid retention and worsen heart failure in an already weak heart when taken in high dosages. Steroids sometimes have an effect on rising blood pressure, especially with high doses. In part, this may be due to sodium retention (see "Water and electrolyte changes" on page 95). Elevated blood pressure improves when steroids are stopped. If steroids are absolutely necessary for asthma treatment, any elevation in blood pressure that may occur can be treated with other medications, such as diuretics, that rid the body of salt.

Infections and Steroids For many years, an increased incidence of infection has been linked with steroids, but this association may not be true.

This is because the association is based on animal studies—where the doses used are a hundred to a thousand times higher than the doses used in humans—and some human diseases that are treated with steroids in themselves predispose to infections.

As a rule, asthmatics taking more than 20 milligrams per day of prednisone over long periods of time seem to be at a slight risk in acquiring infection. On the other hand, individuals taking less than 20 milligrams per day of prednisone or those taking alternate-day steroids even over long periods of time appear to have no increased incidence of infections. *Therefore, the risk of infections from steroids for most asthmatics is minimal.* Infections possibly associated with steroid use usually include fungal infections, such as yeast, athlete's foot, and ringworm; worsening of viral infections, such as chicken pox, shingles, or herpes; and reactivation of tuberculosis.

Side Effects Related to Stopping Steroids   If you are taking prednisone at 10 milligrams (or more) per day for a period of longer than one month, the prednisone can't be stopped abruptly because of possible adrenal gland suppression. This is because the adrenal gland will not "kick in" and make its own steroids when it's supposed to for some time after the prednisone is stopped.

Adrenal gland suppression won't usually happen if the steroid dose is less than 7.5 milligrams per day, if it's taken for less than one month, or if it's taken on alternate days.

Symptoms of adrenal gland suppression consist of loss of appetite, nausea, vomiting, abdominal pain, weakness, and, when severe, falling blood pressure and fever. Symptoms usually occur when there is a stressful event, such as surgery or a major illness, that coincides with stopping the steroids. Most anesthesiologists will give extra steroid medication before surgery to their patients who have taken steroids during the preceding year.

In addition to adrenal gland suppression, another steroid withdrawal syndrome is what's known as pseudorheumatism, which consists of pain and swelling of the joints, localized heat around the joints, and muscle pain, and may last up to 2 weeks. These pseudorheumatism symptoms have no relationship to the dose of and duration of time on the medication. You can usually control these symptoms by using aspirin or other related nonsteroidal anti-inflammatory drugs. (Remember that some asthmatics have aspirin sensitivity and cannot take these drugs; you may need to check with your doctor for substitutes.)

The Most Common Side Effects   We've just discussed *all* the possible side effects associated with steroids. Now we will stress the most common side effects associated with the typical dosage range used in treating asthma. These are:

- increased appetite and weight gain,
- fluid retention,
- increased bruising, and
- mild elevation of blood pressure.

An estimated frequency of these minor side effects occurring in asthma treatment is 25 percent, and all of the side effects reverse when the steroids are discontinued. If steroids are needed to control your asthma and can't be discontinued, the side effects can be minimized with dosage adjustments or other medical intervention. Actually, you could look at these minor side effects as expected effects since they are so frequently experienced when taking steroids.

Side Effects and Form of Treatment   It is important for you to place the side effects of steroids in proper perspective in relationship to the dosage measures and the duration of treatment commonly used for your asthma. Keep in mind that there is a relationship between the side effects of steroids and how often you take them, the dose you take, and the length of time you take them. Precisely, the lower the dose, the less frequently the dose is taken, and the shorter the duration of treatment, the less frequent the side effects. You need to understand these relationships so that you won't become unduly concerned over the side effects of steroids when they are used in treating your asthma.

WHAT YOUR DOCTOR SHOULD KNOW BEFORE YOU TAKE STEROIDS

Tell your doctor if you now have or have had any form of pancreatitis, ulcers, diabetes, osteoporosis, or tuberculosis; any severe cholesterol or tryglyceride abnormalities; or any difficulty with acne, hip injuries, hypertension, herpes, shingles, or myasthenia gravis.

Also, inform your doctor if you are taking other medications:

- diuretics (steroids may increase the loss of potassium with these drugs);
- phenytoin, phenobarbital, ephedrine, or rifampin (all of these drugs decrease the medical effects of steroids);
- oral contraceptives and troleandomycin (these drugs increase the medical effects of steroids);
- aspirin and other nonsteroidal anti-inflammatory agents, such as Indocin, Motrin, Nuprin, Advil, Feldene, Tolectin, Clinoril, Nalfon, Butazolidin, Orudis, Dolobid, and Naprosyn (they increase the incidence of ulcers, and may slightly increase the effects of steroids—for a complete list, see the Glossary); or

- insulin and oral diabetic agents (since steroids increase blood glucose, sometimes more of these medicines will be required to control the increase in blood glucose).

USE OF STEROIDS DURING PREGNANCY

There is no significant evidence that steroids cause adverse effects on the fetus. The indication for use of steroids in asthma is the same for both pregnant and nonpregnant women.

USE OF STEROIDS WHILE NURSING

Steroids appear in breast milk and could possibly reach concentrations high enough to affect the infant. Mothers taking steroids for longer than one month should not nurse.

HABIT-FORMING POTENTIAL OF STEROIDS

None.

EFFECTS OF FOOD, BEVERAGES, AND TOBACCO ON STEROIDS

Food   None.

Nonalcoholic beverages   None.

Alcoholic beverages   None.

Tobacco   None.

INHALED STEROIDS

Inhaled steroids are a minor chemical variation of commonly used oral steroids, which have been synthesized and are used for inhalation in very small doses. These small doses are rapidly metabolized. When inhaled directly into the lungs, they can control asthma without any of the side effects seen with larger doses of orally taken steroids. The potent effect and rapid breakdown in the body of directly inhaled steroids make it possible to take small doses with few side effects.

With regular use of inhaled steroids, a moderate asthmatic can generally control his condition, and only occasionally experience such side effects as yeast infections in the mouth (which can be prevented by rinsing the mouth with water after each inhalation), sore throat, and hoarseness.

Inhaled steroids have some disadvantages: They are not effective in an acute attack of asthma because they do not supply enough steroidal effect to control an acute attack. It's easy to forget to use them since they need to be used several times a day even when you have no symptoms. They are more expensive than most oral steroids. And they are less effective than oral steroids in controlling asthma.

The following table shows some of the names and dosages of inhaled steroids.

Inhaled Steroids

Generic name	Brand name	Dosage
beclomethasone	Vanceril, Beclovent	2 puffs 3–4 times per day
flunisolide	AeroBid	2 puffs 2–3 times per day
triamcinolone	Azmacort	2 puffs 3–4 times per day
budesonide	not commercially available yet	

o   o   o

Learning about the drugs you take will enable you to play a more active role in helping your doctor decide which medical treatment program is safest and most helpful in controlling your asthma. The drugs discussed in this chapter can be used alone, or they may be part of a larger anti-asthma treatment program.

8

Treating and Controlling Your Asthma

By first recognizing and understanding asthma and then by learning about and applying the treatment measures, you'll gain the knowledge that's needed to work effectively along with your doctor in controlling your asthma.

It's possible to control almost all cases of asthma if the right "tools" are used in the right manner. The ultimate goal of asthma treatment is to obtain total remission of your disease. However, when complete remission is not possible, the goal shifts to minimizing your asthma symptoms so that you can live as normally as possible. These goals are achieved through various measures, including:

- medication,
- environmental control,
- allergy shots (immunotherapy), and
- self-help techniques.

Medication

The previous chapter armed you with the basic knowledge and pertinent particulars about *what* medicines are used to treat asthma. Now we will discuss how these medicines are used to effectively treat and control the disease.

Usually medication is the first treatment measure used in asthma, and may be the only measure used in many cases. It's best to take a daily dosage that is convenient and can effectively control your asthma with the least amount of side effects. Some medications seem to be tolerated better than others, depending on the individual asthmatic. For this reason, it may take some time for your doctor to discover which asthma medication works best for you.

The following is an "at-a-glance" view of the medications used in treating and controlling asthma. We've divided them into first-, second-, and third-line medications to let you know the usual manner in which they are used. Following the chart, there's a discussion about how and when to use these drugs.

Medications for Treating and Controlling Asthma

First-line medications	
theophylline	Theophylline drugs can be used intermittently or regularly.
beta stimulators	Beta stimulators can be used with theophylline for additional benefit and (using a hand-held inhaler) quicker relief, or they can be used alone.
Second-line medications	
Cromolyn	Cromolyn can be added and used regularly for asthma not controlled by first-line medications. It's more effective in treating extrinsic asthma.
inhaled steroids	Inhaled steroids can be added and used regularly, alone or with cromolyn, for asthma not controlled by first-line medications.
Third-line medications	
oral steroids	Oral steroids can be used on intermittent, short courses for flare-ups of asthma. Prolonged daily or alternate-day steroids can be used for severe, chronic asthma.

One "first-line" drug in treating asthma is theophylline. Any number of theophylline preparations listed in the previous chapter can be prescribed by your doctor.

It's important for asthmatics to start taking theophylline as soon as their symptoms (coughing, wheezing, shortness of breath) begin; this will prevent the asthma from snowballing into a severe attack. As the windpipes narrow, they become more sensitive to additional asthma triggers; keeping the windpipes open with early treatment lessens their sensitivity to these triggers. When you first take theophylline, it takes several hours to reach a therapeutic blood level (the blood level at which drugs work most effectively). This is another reason it's important to start taking theophylline as soon as your symptoms begin.

Chronic asthmatics generally take "long-acting" (time-released) theophylline preparations, whereas those with acute asthma may take "short-acting" theophylline preparations because they work quicker. Depending on the activity of your asthma, your doctor will decide whether theophylline should be used on a regular basis (all the time) or intermittently (when needed). Your doctor may want to monitor theophylline concentrations to prevent toxicity or to improve control of your asthma if the originally selected dosage isn't adequately controlling your symptoms. This is usually done by a blood test after you've taken four or five doses.

It's often incorrectly recommended to take theophylline with food on the premise that the drug may upset your stomach. Unfortunately, taking theophylline with food may decrease its absorption, allowing less medicine to get into your blood stream. A little food won't interfere, but it's not a good idea to have a large meal.

Beta stimulators are another type of "first-line" drug used for asthma. They may be as important as theophylline in controlling asthma. They can be taken with theophylline when daily symptoms can't be controlled with theophylline alone. Because beta stimulators work in a different way than theophylline to open the windpipes, they can have an additive effect to the action of theophylline. Sometimes beta stimulators are used alone by asthmatics who can't tolerate theophylline, and they may be used alone in hand-held inhalers by some people who have occasional asthma attacks. Usually adults prefer inhaled beta stimulators over those taken by mouth because they work quicker and cause less nervousness. However, children often find them difficult to use, so oral beta stimulators are usually a better alternative for them. Sometimes when severe attacks occur frequently with young children, a motorized nebulizer can be helpful. This allows the parent to give the child a nebulized treatment (mist treatment inhaled by mouth) of a beta-stimulator medication and get rapid improvement. Nebulized treatment may cut down on trips to hospital emergency rooms to treat the child's severe asthma attacks.

There are small adaptors for hand-held inhalers available under the names, Inhal-Aid, Inspirease, and Aero-Chamber. These adaptors make it easier for children to use hand-held inhalers by eliminating the need to time the inhalation with the delivery of medicine. In some cases, these adaptors may be as effective as the motorized nebulizer in treating acute asthma attacks.

As with theophylline, it's best to use beta stimulators when symptoms first begin to prevent the asthma from snowballing into a severe attack.

It is important to take beta stimulators *as directed* by your doctor every 4 to 8 hours, depending on the preparation. It's best to divide doses as equally spaced as possible throughout 24 hours. Depending on the activity of your asthma, your doctor will decide whether beta stimulators should be used on a regular basis or intermittently.

When symptoms can't be controlled by "first-line" medications (theophylline or beta stimulators), a trial use of cromolyn may be helpful, especially if you are an extrinsic asthmatic. Cromolyn doesn't work as a bronchodilator as does theophylline or beta stimulators, but controls asthma by *preventing* bronchospasms.

It's important to take cromolyn *as directed* by your doctor. The dosage should be spaced as far apart as conveniently possible while you're awake—for instance, first thing in the morning, after school or work, after dinner, and at bedtime.

Cromolyn should never be used during an existing asthma attack because its powdery substance will further irritate the windpipes, and it has no beneficial effect on an existing attack. To be effective, you must use it prior to being exposed to an asthma trigger; therefore, you must use it on a regular basis as a preventive measure.

Cromolyn is always taken by inhalation (it's also available in a solution for the motorized nebulizer). It would have no benefit if taken by mouth because it isn't absorbed well by the gastrointestinal tract.

Another group of medications that can be used as a preventive measure are inhaled steroids. As with cromolyn, these medicines must also be used on a regular basis—even when you have no symptoms—and they are not effective during an acute asthma attack.

Inhaled steroids can be used along with cromolyn, theophylline, and beta stimulators. They are best suited for controlling chronic, moderate asthma. Inhaled steroids can also be helpful when used along with oral steroids for treating chronic, severe asthma because they will allow you to take lower oral steroid doses and still get good control.

If your asthma isn't controlled well by any of the "first- and second-line" medications, you should use oral steroids. Oral steroids should be taken *as directed* by your doctor. There are many different ways to take them, depending on the severity of your asthma, how long it has lasted, and how well you've responded to other medications.

Prednisone is the most common steroid used. It is usually taken at a relatively high dose two times a day at the beginning; then the dose is tapered over the subsequent 7 to 10 days, depending on the response. After 10 days, it may be discontinued. However, sometimes doctors will want to continue prednisone on a low-dose alternate-day basis for about one month because after an asthma attack the airways may remain more reactive to additional asthma triggers for several weeks.

If your asthma is severe and/or chronic, it may require prolonged oral steroid treatment for control. When prolonged oral steroids are needed to control asthma, the lower the dose, the safer—and alternate-day doses are safer than daily doses. Generally, the short-acting steroids, such as prednisone and methylprednisolone, are safer than long-acting steroids. If your asthma is very severe, you may require high-dose daily steroids for long periods of time, which may bring on considerable side effects. (See Chapter 7 for more information about side effects.)

Recently, the use of troleandomycin (Tao), an antibiotic, taken in low doses in conjunction with methylprednisolone (not prednisone), has been effective in helping the steroid dose to be lowered and/or changed to alternate-day doses while still obtaining maximal control of severe asthma.

If you have used prednisone on a daily basis for longer than one month, it needs to be slowly tapered off rather than stopped abruptly. Daily use of prednisone for longer than one month suppresses the adrenal gland's ability to produce its own steroids. Therefore, prednisone needs to be slowly tapered to let the adrenal gland start making its own steroids.

You don't need to taper the prednisone dose before stopping it in two instances:

- when used daily for less than one month or
- when used on an alternate-day basis for any length of time.

In these situations, there is little suppression of the adrenal gland's ability to make its own steroids.

To ensure there will be no adrenal gland suppression when prednisone is taken on an alternate-day basis, it should be taken in the morning.

You shouldn't stop taking prednisone just because your symptoms subside; always take this medicine until your doctor says to stop.

Asthma can be categorized as mild, moderate, or severe, and occurs in an intermittent or chronic manner (for category definitions, see "Asthma, Classifications of " in the Glossary). How your asthma is categorized determines what medicine you should use and how it should be taken. The following "at-a-glance" table can be helpful in these decisions. However, it's still important to check with your doctor.

Methods for Taking Asthma Drugs

Mild Intermittent
Use theophylline *or* inhaled or oral beta stimulators on an "as-needed" basis.

Moderate Intermittent
Use theophylline *in addition to* inhaled or oral beta stimulators on an "as-needed" basis.

Severe Intermittent
Use theophylline in addition to inhaled or oral beta stimulators on an "as-

needed" basis. If attacks are frequent, continuous use of inhaled steroids and/or inhaled cromolyn will help prevent attacks. Short courses of prednisone are often necessary.

Mild Chronic

Use "long-acting" theophylline regularly. Add inhaled or oral beta stimulators for asthma flare-ups.

Moderate Chronic

Use "long-acting" theophylline regularly. Add inhaled or oral beta stimulators for asthma flare-ups. If problem persists, add inhaled cromolyn and/or inhaled steroids on a regular basis. Short courses of prednisone are often necessary for acute asthma flare-ups.

Severe Chronic

Use "long-acting" theophylline regularly. Use inhaled or oral beta stimulators regularly. Use inhaled cromolyn and/or inhaled steroids regularly. The regular use of alternate-day or daily low-dose prednisone is often needed.

People often wonder if antibiotics are effective in treating asthma, especially because infections are a major trigger for asthma attacks. Since almost all infection triggers for asthma are viruses, antibiotics are usually of no benefit. However, there are some circumstances in which antibiotics are beneficial:

- Occasionally mycoplasma, an antibiotic-sensitive germ that is not a virus, can trigger asthma, and is treated with erythromycin;
- Sinusitis (bacterial), which is frequently associated with asthma and may trigger asthma symptoms, is treated with antibiotics; and
- Other associated bacterial infections, such as pneumonia or otitis media (ear infection), require antibiotics.

Another common question people often have involves the use of flu vaccines in the treatment of asthma. Since influenza infection is a major trigger for severe asthma attacks, flu shots are helpful. Some asthmatics experience a mild increase in asthma symptoms after receiving a flu shot, but these symptoms are very minor compared to the severe asthma attacks that may be triggered by a flu infection.

Sometimes antihistamines are tried in the treatment of asthma, but they have little or no beneficial effect, especially since many other internal chemicals besides histamine affect asthma. However, antihistamines are helpful for asthma-associated nasal conditions, such as allergic rhinitis.

Warnings on various antihistamine medications declaring their possible hazards to asthmatics are simply not true. Antihistamines can be used to treat nasal conditions in an asthmatic.

A new class of drugs that are effective as bronchodilators have been used in Europe for several years. They are known as anticholinergic drugs. The first of this kind of drug has recently been released in the United States, and is called ipratropium bromide, or Atrovent. It works by blocking the cholinergic part of the nervous system to the windpipes. By blocking this part of the nervous system, it causes bronchodilatation. Presently this drug is used for its airway-opening abilities more with bronchitis than with asthma. This is because generally, with asthma, the beta stimulators work better than ipratropium and other known anticholinergic drugs. However, some asthmatics may respond better to anticholinergic drugs. Eventually, more effective drugs in this class may be developed and ultimately used for asthma.

Presently ipratropium bromide (Atrovent) is available in a hand-held inhaler and is taken by inhaling two puffs four times per day.

Environmental Control

Environmental control measures, sometimes referred to as avoidance measures, are aimed at minimizing exposure to known allergens in your living and working environments. By minimizing your exposure to asthma triggers, you minimize your asthma symptoms. For this reason, environmental control is considered an important measure in controlling asthma, especially extrinsic (allergic) asthma.

An ideal goal for environmental control would be total elimination of all asthmatic triggers. But no one can live life in a sterile bubble; such an existence would be neither desirable nor practical. Rather than total elimination of allergens, a more realistic goal would be to minimize exposure to as many asthma triggers as possible. To achieve this, you must be aware of which allergens trigger your asthma. Awareness enables you to avoid the troublesome triggers and control your environment to some workable degree.

For some asthmatics, knowing what triggers their symptoms is obvious. For the asthmatic who wheezes only when encountering cats or the asthmatic who wheezes only upon entering a damp mould-infested basement, detecting the cause of his symptoms is certainly no mystery. Likewise, recognizing offending allergens is fairly simple for the asthmatic who wheezes whenever he sleeps on a feather pillow or for the asthmatic who wheezes only during a particular pollinating season. Unfortunately, for most asthmatics, crystal-clear identification of triggering allergens is not this easy, especially if their asthma is chronic throughout most of the year. For this reason, allergy skin testing becomes necessary to confirm allergic triggers suspected by the asthmatic and to uncover additional, unsuspected triggering culprits. Results of skin testing aid in pinpointing allergic triggers and thus in initiating subsequent environmental control measures.

HOW MUCH ENVIRONMENTAL CONTROL SHOULD AN ASTHMATIC UNDERTAKE?

If your physician determines that environmental control measures would be advantageous in combating your particular asthma, you should approach this means of control as vigorously as you can. The amount of environmental control you should undertake depends upon five factors:

- the type of allergen and the ease of avoidance of that allergen,

- the severity of your allergy and asthma,

- your motivation and the time you have available to undertake environmental control measures,

- your financial resources available for carrying out some of the more specific environmental control measures (such as special air filters), and

- how well other types of treatment (drugs and allergy shots) are working to control your asthma.

Let's examine each of these five factors more closely:

- It's virtually impossible to avoid exposure to some allergens, such as pollens, because they are everywhere. Likewise, if a person's occupation exposes him to an offending allergen (as is the case with a veterinarian working with cats and dogs or a golf pro working around grass), then controlling exposure to the allergen becomes nearly impossible.

- If an individual's asthma is severe and his allergy to the trigger is severe, it may be necessary for him to go to greater lengths in environmental control measures to help control his asthma.

- Some asthmatics simply don't have enough motivation to put forth the effort to control their environment. Some people don't have the time to take the necessary steps to control their environment. And some asthmatics refuse to give up a favorite pet or other part of their lives that gives them comfort or pleasure even though it provokes their asthma.

- Some environmental control measures require the use of expensive equipment, such as air conditioners and air filters or other such paraphernalia. It may be difficult for some people to find the financial resources to provide for these measures.

- At times, asthmatics do well on medication alone without experiencing any side effects, and thus find it unnecessary to take on environmental control measures. Also, some asthmatics can achieve control with allergy shots without the use of environmental control measures.

If you feel you would benefit from environmental control, concentrate on the areas and places where you spend most of your time. Most people spend the majority of their time in the bedroom; in fact, about one-third of their time is spent in the bedroom. Other important areas to check for allergen exposure are your favorite rooms in your home, your car, and your workplace. If your child has asthma, check his school or day-care environment. Start your control measures by focusing on the allergens that bother you the most and are the easiest to control.

WHAT ALLERGENS ARE SUITABLE FOR ENVIRONMENTAL CONTROL ?

Dust Although you can't achieve a completely "dust-free" environment, you can obtain a "dust-poor" environment if you try. Ideally, a "dust-poor" room should contain a minimal amount of furniture, which is not cluttered with dust-collecting knickknacks so that it's easy to clean. You should avoid having heavy drapes and upholstered items because they collect and hold dust. If possible, try to avoid having carpeting since it requires vacuuming, which stirs up and scatters dust particles into the environment. Hardwood and tile flooring, on the other hand, can be damp-mopped, which diminishes the scattering of dust.

Dust control in your bedroom is of primary importance since you spend so much time there. You can accomplish dust control in the bedroom by encasing box-spring mattresses in a dust-proof vinyl cover. Then place a mattress pad over the vinyl to guard against irritation and to ensure greater sleeping comfort. Covering your mattress this way retards the spread of dust from the mattress and the growth of dust mites, which thrive in the warm, moist environment created by your body resting on the mattress. Dust mites feed off human dander, which you naturally shed onto your mattress. By acting as a barrier between you and the mattress, the cover reduces the amount of human dander shed onto the mattress. Another way to gain control is by using a smooth-finish bedspread as opposed to a chenille type with a bumpy surface. Bumpy-surfaced bedspreads are dust catchers. Remove other dust catchers, such as stuffed animals, books, and stored clothing. A thorough weekly cleaning contributes to a "dust-poor" environment, as does daily dusting. Using dust-settling compounds on your dust cloth or dust mop helps to "trap" dust. While these measures may be time-consuming, they are worth the effort if they can reduce your exposure to the triggers that provoke your asthma.

Tremendously helpful aids when dust allergy is severe are special air filters, called electrostatic precipitators. They filter the air very effectively, and can be applied to a central-heating unit or used alone as a portable unit. Their range of efficiency for removing particles—such as dust, pollens, moulds, and other allergens and irritants—from the air is 70 to 90 percent. One possible drawback with these air filters is that they have the potential of producing ozone, which in turn may trigger asthma because of its irritant effect. However, this usually isn't a problem unless the ozone is great enough to cause an odor and is in close proximity to the asthmatic.

Another high-efficiency filter is what's known as a HEPA filter (high efficiency particulate air filter). It is generally used as a portable unit, and presently is not well suited to central-heating units. Ranked as one of the most efficient air cleaners available, it has an extended surface composed of microscopic glass and asbestos fibres, which renders it capable of removing 99 percent of all particles from the air. It effectively removes fumes, aerosols, dust, smoke, pollens, moulds, and even bacteria from the environment. It's best to place HEPA filters near the head of your bed, where the air flow, a few feet from the back side of the filter, would be almost 100 percent clear of allergens and irritants.

Moulds

Indoor moulds To control indoor mould, dampness must be eliminated as much as possible. The use of electric heaters or dehumidifiers can cut down on dampness and reduce mould growth, especially in damp basements. The use of louvred doors, ventilation holes, and a burning light bulb can be helpful in reducing moisture in damp closets. Window sills and shower stalls are good growing grounds for moulds. To discourage mould growth, wipe them down or scrub them briskly with a brush using a fungicidal solution, such as Lysol or Clorox. Walls can facilitate mould growth, too; however, you can prevent this by keeping beds, dressers, and other furniture about 6 inches away from them to allow for greater air circulation. In addition, all rooms should be properly ventilated to inhibit moisture formation. Crawl spaces should be completely covered with plastic sheeting to prevent mould spores in the moist ground from rising into your house. Removing houseplants may be necessary since their potted soil and dead leaves provide nourishment for moulds. In addition, a HEPA filter may be helpful in removing mould spores from the air.

If you are plagued by severe mould problems that can't be resolved by these control measures, you may need to resort to chemical fumigation. To fumigate a room or closet, place one of the following chemical fumigants within it:

- formaldehyde solution ($\frac{1}{2}$ to 1 pint) in a shallow vessel or
- crystals of paraformaldehyde (trioxymethylene) ($\frac{1}{2}$ ounce) in a wide-mouth jar.

Then close off the room or closet for a week. Formaldehyde fumes are irritating to the nose and lungs, but won't harm wood finishes, wallpaper, or fabrics unless spilled directly on them. At the end of the fumigation, the room or closet should be well ventilated and allowed to air out before anyone with asthma or other respiratory problems uses it.

Outdoor moulds Outdoor moulds can be controlled to a certain degree. To foil the invasion of mould spores into your home, close your windows and/or use a window air conditioner, particularly in the bedroom and especially during the more troublesome times of the year. Grass and leaves have a heavy mould growth. Mowing and raking disturbs this heavy mould growth, causing the spores to become airborne which consequently wreaks havoc on those who are allergic to mould. For the same reasons, mold-allergic children shouldn't frolic in the leaves and stir up the mould spores. To further control outdoor moulds, eliminate any vines and shrubs that may be growing against the walls of your house, remove all dead leaves from your yard, and avoid compost piles. In general, outdoor moulds are as difficult to control as pollens. You can't remove mould-spore sources in the outdoor environment, but you can minimize your exposure.

Animal Danders The degree of animal-dander allergy varies from person to person. For some, reduced contact with the animal may be all that is needed to control asthma symptoms; for others, total elimination of the animal from the environment may be the only answer. In most cases, keeping the animal outdoors is sufficient. Limited time indoors for the animal may be all right, although animal dander can be spread throughout the house by forced-air heating systems, even when the animal is allowed in the house for short periods of time or limited to one place. Therefore, when someone has a severe animal sensitivity, exposure should be eliminated altogether.

Even after the animal is removed from the house, the allergen may persist in the environment for months. For this reason, a thorough house-cleaning is recommended. Also, a child may be exposed to animals at a babysitter's home or at school, or other family members may be in constant contact with animals; they will inevitably bring animal dander in on their clothing, which will invade your environment and possibly cause allergic symptoms.

If you are sensitive to a particular animal species, you are usually sensitive to all varieties of that species. Don't get caught up in the misconceived notion that only some dogs and cats are allergenic. This simply is not true.

Pollen You cannot effectively remove pollen sources in the outdoor environment. But, obviously, adults and children who are sensitive to weed, grass, and/or tree pollens shouldn't work or play in fields or areas abundant in these allergens.

On the other hand, you can control the degree to which pollen enters your home. Close your windows during bothersome pollinating seasons. For greater control in your bedroom, a window air-conditioning unit is helpful in filtering pollen from the air. Central air conditioning is ideal for the whole house, but it's often very expensive because of increasing electrical rates.

Other Allergens Feather pillows are highly allergenic to some people, not only because of their feather allergen, but because they also contain abundant dust-mite and mould allergens. Pillows should be encased in nonallergenic covers. While dust-proof pillow covers act as a barrier between your own dander and dust-mite growth, they don't prevent feather allergens from leaking out; so your best move would be to replace feather pillows with nonallergenic pillows made of dacron or polyester. Don't replace them with foam-rubber pillows because they support mould growth. Also, it's important to avoid all other sources of feathers—such as down sleeping bags, jackets, or bed comforters.

You can easily avoid cottonseed, kapok, and flaxseed by steering clear of the sleeping bags, furniture, and stuffed animals that may be stuffed with these allergens.

If you are susceptible to jute allergen, stay away from jute-back carpeting or hobbies involving macramé.

If you're allergic to wool, replace all woollen products with products made of other materials. If other members of your family have woollen garments, store them in plastic garment bags to prevent their particles from entering your environment.

If you happen to be allergic to pyrethrum, avoid insecticides which contain this substance. Pyrethrum is an allergen that is similar to ragweed; so if you have ragweed allergy, it may help to steer clear of insecticides containing pyrethrum.

WHAT NONALLERGENIC IRRITANTS SHOULD BE CONTROLLED?

Irritating substances are nonallergenic sources of asthma triggers. Outside irritants are difficult to control, but indoor irritants can be minimized. Smoking, a tremendous irritant that exacerbates both upper- and lower-respiratory-tract problems, should be prohibited inside the asthmatic's home and car. Various other irritants—such as perfumes, hair sprays, and other volatile substances that produce strong odors—should be avoided.

Likewise, kerosene heaters shouldn't be used around the asthmatic because their fumes contain sulfur dioxide and are emitted in concentrations that can easily produce asthma symptoms. Woodburning stoves, if improperly installed, can cause fumes and soot to leak into the environment, which may trigger asthma symptoms.

SHOULD AN ASTHMATIC MOVE TO ANOTHER ENVIRONMENT TO GAIN GREATER CONTROL OF HIS CONDITION?

Rarely is geographic relocation advocated or encouraged as a workable control measure for an asthmatic. Should a severe asthmatic be plagued by long, intense seasonal pollen exposures and consider moving, he would need to weigh the desirable medical benefits of geographic relocation against the inevitable psychological, social, and financial changes that such a move would present to him and his family. Also, it's important to realize that frequently after a move, an asthmatic may experience short-term improvement, but then his symptoms gradually recur as he becomes sensitive to allergens in the new environment. However, moves away from certain environmental irritants, such as factories that permeate the surrounding air with pollutants, can be beneficial for some asthmatics, and do not require total geographic relocation.

It's best to take a common sense approach to environmental control. You and your doctor must ultimately decide the amount of environmental control that would be the most beneficial for your individual condition.

In spite of employing good environmental control measures and using proper medications, some asthmatics may continue to have difficulty controlling their symptoms. For these people, immunotherapy may be a necessary part of their treatment.

Immunotherapy

Immunotherapy, or allergy shots, is a treatment whereby a person receives injections of a substance to which he is allergic in an attempt to reduce his sensitivity to that substance. Two other terms used for immunotherapy are hyposensitization and desensitization.

Immunotherapy has been used as a form of treatment in one modification or another since 1911. Since 1960, laboratory technology has been able to determine the best procedure and dose for allergy shots as well as the types of allergy that get the best results from them.

An asthmatic takes various skin tests to discover his specific allergens. From their results, an allergist can prepare an allergy-shot preparation. The asthmatic takes allergy shots every 3 to 7 days, beginning with small doses and then building up to large doses. As time passes, the asthmatic graduates to a maintenance dose, which he takes every 3 to 4 weeks for about 4 years.

The best results obtained from allergy shots occur in individuals with allergies to pollen (especially ragweed and grass), house dust, and some animal danders. Allergy shots for mould allergy are less effective, but some allergists believe that prolonged treatment with allergy shots (more than 4 years) does result in significant clinical improvement in asthmatics with mould allergy.

Allergy shots are not effective against bacteria; most chemicals; foods; and extracts of nonprotein materials—such as nylon, Kleenex, and newsprint, to name a few.

Allergy shots are usually necessary when:

- allergy is an important trigger for asthma,
- the allergy is one that will respond to immunotherapy, and
- symptoms continue despite reasonable environmental control and use of asthma medications.

Allergy shots, as opposed to treatment with drugs alone, offers the asthmatic a chance for long-term improvement. Decisions regarding allergy shots should be made by a well-trained allergist familiar with the complexities of diagnosis, the techniques of immunotherapy, and the other available alternate therapies for the treatment of asthma.

HOW DO ALLERGY SHOTS WORK IN TREATING ASTHMA?

How allergy shots work is not completely known. We do know that several immunologic events occur in someone receiving allergy shots, and when these events occur, the asthma symptoms seem to improve.

Allergy shots reduce the amount of histamine released during an allergic reaction, and they also decrease the amount of IgE allergic antibody. These two events seem to play the most important roles in decreasing allergic asthma symptoms.

With allergy shots, another kind of antibody—IgG—increases. It works as a "blocking antibody" and neutralizes allergens. Increasing the IgG "blocking" antibody is important because it allows the asthmatic to take and tolerate allergy shots in larger and larger doses.

WHAT ADVERSE REACTIONS ARE ASSOCIATED WITH ALLERGY SHOTS?

Reactions to allergy shots can be local or systemic. Local reactions aren't very significant, but can cause considerable discomfort. A local reaction will manifest as an itchy, raised, reddened area around the injection site. It can usually be treated with antihistamines, aspirin, and ice packs, if necessary. If a white wheal greater than the size of a quarter should develop within 15 to 20 minutes of your injection, the dosage of your next shot may have to stay the same or be decreased. Local reactions may also occur several hours to one day after the injection; even though they are red, swollen, and sometimes painful, these delayed reactions are of no serious consequence and don't require a dosage adjustment for the next shot.

Systemic reactions are serious and, in rare instances, can be fatal. They may consist of symptoms of asthma, along with nasal congestion and a runny nose. Also, general itching, hives, flushing, nausea, vomiting, diarrhea, fullness in the throat, and fainting may occur in systemic reactions. If treated properly with adrenaline and antihistamines, they can be rapidly controlled in almost all instances. Systemic reactions are not very common when allergy shots are administered correctly. When they do occur, your next shot dosage must be decreased.

To observe for reactions, you should wait at least 20 minutes in your physician's office after you receive your allergy shot. Severe systemic reactions usually occur within 20 minutes. However, milder systemic reactions may occur up to 2 to 3 hours after a shot.

ARE ALLERGY SHOTS ALWAYS SUCCESSFUL?

When you receive allergy shots, you should expect about a 75 percent improvement in about 2 to 3 years. Sometimes allergy shots aren't successful. Some reasons may be:

- inaccurate allergy testing,
- use of allergy shots for intrinsic (nonallergic) asthma,
- new allergens developing after the shots have been started,
- use of inadequate dosages and injection schedules for the allergy shots, or
- failure of the allergy shots to cause the necessary immunologic changes in the body that will result in improvement.

ARE SOME IMMUNOTHERAPY TECHNIQUES CONTROVERSIAL?

When you are looking for allergic control of your asthma, you will discover that all physicians do not subscribe to the same practices and techniques. In fact, certain testing and treatment techniques have become quite controversial. In 1981, the American Academy of Allergy made a position statement regarding several of these techniques. It maintained that:

- the Rinkel method of skin testing—which is used for determining a starting and maintenance allergy-shot dose—is generally inaccurate,
- subcutaneous testing to provoke and neutralize symptoms as a method for diagnosing and treating allergic diseases has no validity, and
- sublingual (drops of allergens under the tongue) testing is not valid and sublingual treatment results in no improvements.

These controversial techniques are discussed in greater detail in Chapter 5.

A controversial surgical procedure that, its proponents profess, aids in treating asthma is *bilateral carotid body resection*. The carotid bodies are located near the carotid arteries on both sides of the neck. They are important in controlling a person's amount of breathing. The surgery removes these breathing sensors and, as a result, the asthma is supposed to improve. However, this procedure has never been shown to be effective in treating asthma, and carries with it a significant mortality rate.

Self-Help Techniques

Chest Physiotherapy   This includes postural drainage and chest percussion, which can help clear mucous secretions from your lungs. They are done by lying on your stomach over the side of a bed and extending your chest and head to the floor. Have a partner "clap" up and down on your back directly behind your chest with cupped hands for about 5 minutes. This produces a hollow sound and causes just enough vibration to shake loose the mucus in your lungs so that you can easily cough it up.

Breathing-Control Exercises   These exercises teach you how to do relaxed breathing. Most asthmatics tend to hyperventilate, especially if they're under stress. Hyperventilation frequently causes increased discomfort by making the shortness of breath often associated with asthma actually much worse. Relaxed-breathing exercises allow you to control the hyperventilation problem. (For more information about self-help techniques for controlling hyperventilation, see Chapter 15.)

Breathing-Muscle Training Exercises   There are a host of exercises that are supposed to improve the strength of your breathing muscles, but they take time and are of questionable benefit. However, recently, inspiratory muscle trainers have become available. These small devices are designed to increase the strength and endurance of the respiratory muscle. While you inhale through it, the device provides resistance to make your respiratory muscles work harder. As with any exercise, you must practise this routinely for best results.

Special Exercises for Children   Blowing up balloons, blowing bubbles, blowing Ping Pong balls across a table, and blowing on a musical instrument are all good and enjoyable breathing exercises for children, and may improve their breathing capacity.

o   o   o

In the last few chapters, you have discovered the series of steps that can lead you from diagnosis to treatment of your condition. Ideally, you and your doctor are teammates in conquering your asthma. He provides insight into the diagnosis and treatment techniques of asthma, and you provide help by relating your signs and symptoms of asthma as well as your suspected asthma triggers. With his help, you can gain invaluable knowledge about your condition; with your help, he can gain invaluable knowledge about you and your particular circumstances, which will help him establish the best individualized treatment program for you. Together, the two of you can rely on each other to recognize and treat symptoms of asthma *before* they get out of control.

Triumph over your condition can be exciting and rewarding; it can give you a sense of control over an important area of your life—your health care. And with control, you have the ability and power to enhance the quality of your life.

9
Surgery, Anesthesia, and Asthma

Surgery and anesthesia present special problems for the asthmatic. Of all asthmatics, 5.6 percent will develop asthma attacks during surgery, and extrinsic (allergic) asthmatics are at an increased risk of allergic reactions to anesthesia. Of all complications in asthmatics during or after surgery, 75 percent are related to the respiratory system. However, these problems can be lessened or prevented with proper planning and precautionary measures.

What Can I Do Before Surgery To Lessen Problems?
The most important thing you should do is tell your surgeon and anesthesiologist you are asthmatic. You should also give them a general idea of the last time you had symptoms, and accurately detail the medications you are taking to control your asthma. You will need to relate any conditions, such as heartbeat irregularities, which can be complicated by the combination of asthma medicines and anesthesia. It's also important to:

- avoid smoking (even passive smoke) for at least one week prior to surgery since smoking aggravates asthma by causing bronchospasm and interfering with your windpipes' ability to clear secretions;

- take extra precaution not to catch a cold one month prior to surgery since a cold can increase your chance of developing asthma during anesthesia (colds cause increased windpipe hyperreactivity);

- drink more water the day before surgery to counteract the drying effects anesthesia has on windpipes;

- practise relaxed-breathing techniques (see Chapter 15) to control your breathing, thereby avoiding anxiety, hyperventilation, and worsening your asthma; and

• tell your doctor about any medications to which you are allergic, such as aspirin and other nonsteroidal anti-inflammatory drugs, or penicillin.

What Will My Doctor Need To Do Before Surgery?

The most important thing your doctor will need to do before surgery is assess your present asthma condition. He does this by giving you a physical exam and, if needed, pulmonary function and blood gas tests. These measures are also used to determine the appropriate anesthetic agents best suited for you and to prepare for any complications during and after surgery.

Before surgery, your doctor may treat any complicating infections, such as a sinus infection or other upper- and lower-respiratory infections. He also may treat you with asthma medicines before surgery, if necessary. Maximum control of asthma is important prior to surgery to prevent the development of asthma during and after surgery and to prevent any other postoperative respiratory complications.

Sometimes surgery is an emergency and preoperative plans can't be made as well as one would like. But even then, with the proper selection of preoperative medications, muscle relaxants, anesthesia-inducing agents, and general anesthetic agents for maintenance, your asthma can still be well controlled and result in no increased complications.

How Can Asthma Medicines Affect Surgery and Anesthesia?

If you routinely need asthma medications to control your asthma, you'll need to continue them up to the time of surgery, during surgery, and after surgery to lessen the chances of anesthesia and surgery worsening your asthma. The following are descriptions of how the most common asthma medications can affect surgery and anesthesia.

Theophylline Theophylline may cause heartbeat irregularities when taken along with halothane, a drug commonly used for general anesthesia. Your doctor will want to make sure your theophylline dose is proper for a blood level in the therapeutic range before surgery.

Beta Stimulators Since beta stimulators can cause heartbeat irregularities when taken with halothane, you should use the smallest dose to control your asthma. It's better to use inhaled beta stimulators at this time because they have less of an effect on the heart than equivalent doses of oral beta stimulators.

Steroids The use of steroids can cause suppression of the adrenal gland.

The stress response during and after surgery requires the adrenal gland to produce steroids in large amounts. This helps your body adjust to the stressful event. If you have taken more than the equivalent of 7.5 milligrams per day of prednisone for longer than one month during the past year, there may be some adrenal suppression. Therefore, you need to take supplemental steroids just before and after surgery to compensate for the adrenal gland's inability to make enough steroids. If you've taken high doses (more than 10 milligrams per day) for some time (longer than 3 months), an additional problem may occur—your skin may become thinner, resulting in slower healing after surgery.

What Are My Options in Anesthesia for Surgery?

There are two types of anesthesia—local and general.

Local anesthesia is caused by the injection of anesthetic agents directly into the surgical area or into nerves supplying the surgical area. There are four kinds of local anesthetics:

- direct (injecting the anesthetic agent just under the skin to provide a numbing effect), used in oral surgery and for removal of superficial skin lesions;
- nerve block (injecting the anesthetic agent into the nerve that supplies the surgical area), most commonly used to anesthetize arms or legs for surgery and to numb the birth canal for delivery;
- spinal (injecting the anesthetic agent directly into the spinal canal), most commonly used for lower-abdominal or leg surgery or for obstetrics; and
- epidural (injecting the anesthetic just outside the spinal canal lining), used for lower-abdominal surgery or obstetrics.

General anesthesia is caused by the loss of consciousness under a controlled setting. It is usually induced by injecting a drug (inducting agent) and then maintained by inhaling an anesthetic gas. Intubation (insertion of a tube into the windpipes to give the anesthesiologist access to the airways for breathing support) is usually necessary during general anesthesia, especially if the surgery is extensive and prolonged.

How Does Anesthesia Affect Asthma?

With the possible exception of spinal anesthesia, local anesthesia usually has no adverse effects on the asthmatic. If the spinal anesthesia is used high up in the spine for abdominal surgery, it may block important chemicals, such as epinephrine, from being released by the adrenal gland. Epinephrine is necessary for internal control of asthma; if its release is blocked, asthma symptoms may occur.

General anesthesia may have adverse effects on asthma in two ways:
- from drugs used in obtaining general anesthesia and
- from intubation, which may irritate the airways and cause bronchospasm (this is the major cause of asthma aggravation during surgery).

What Drugs Are Used Before, During, and After Surgery?

Preoperative Medications Common medications include diazepam (Valium), midazolam (Versed), morphine, meperidine (Demerol), and fentanyl (Sublimaze). Which drugs are used depends on the anesthesiologist's preference. Meperidine and morphine can cause the release of histamine and can aggravate asthma.

Muscle-Relaxing Agents These medications are used to assist in intubation at the time of general anesthesia. Some muscle relaxants are pancuronium, succinylcholine, and tubocurarine. Although all are considered safe for asthmatics, pancuronium is favored because it never causes histamine release and ensuing bronchospasm.

Anesthetic-Inducing Agents Common agents include thiopental (Pentothal), methohexital (Brevitol), and ketamine (Ketalar). Thiopenthal and methohexital both can cause bronchospasm, but methohexital is less likely to do so. Ketamine does not cause bronchospasm.

Anesthetic-Maintenance Agents These gas anesthetics include halothane, enflurane, insoflurane, methoxyflurane, nitrous oxide, cyclopropane, ethylene, and ether. Cyclopropane, ethylene, and ether are rarely used anymore because they are flammable and the safer anesthetics are preferred. Halothane is considered the anesthetic of choice for asthmatics because of its bronchodilating effect and because it doesn't cause windpipe irritation or mucous formation. Halothane aggravates the irregular heartbeat effects of asthma drugs, however. Enflurane and isoflurane are newer anesthetics that also cause bronchodilation but do not cause irregular heartbeats.

Postoperative Medications The same medications used preoperatively for sedation and analgesia are often used postoperatively. Diazepam and midazolam are commonly used for sedation, whereas morphine, meperidine, and fentanyl are used for pain relief. Meperidine and morphine can cause the release of histamine and aggravate asthma. All of these medications can suppress respiration and interfere with the coughing reflex. Your doctor may want to limit the dose of these drugs if you're asthmatic.

What Postoperative Complications Involve the Respiratory System?

Respiratory system complications are more common with upper-abdominal and thoracic procedures than with lower-abdominal and extremity surgery. This is especially true with asthmatics. Respiratory complications occur because the pain of surgery and the use of postoperative medicines interfere with your ability to cough and clear secretions from your windpipes, thereby decreasing normal ventilation. This can cause atelectasis (collapse of certain areas of the lung), pneumonia (lung infection), and worsening of asthma symptoms. Each of these can result in low blood-oxygen levels and a major problem for you postoperatively.

What Can I and My Doctor Do To Prevent Postoperative Complications?

You should cough as much as possible to keep your windpipes clear of mucous secretions. Also, take deep breaths to prevent atelectasis. Sometimes asthmatics use a device, called an incentive spirometer, to encourage deep breathing and to monitor the amount and effect of their efforts. Additionally, practising the relaxed-breathing techniques discussed in Chapter 15 can help you control the stress and hyperventilation, caused by the pain of surgery, that aggravate asthma.

Your doctor may give you beta stimulators in a warm saline solution by inhalation along with intravenous aminophylline to prevent or control your asthma. He also may want a respiratory therapist to give you chest physiotherapy (cupped hand clapping applied to the chest area) to help you loosen and get rid of the mucous secretions from your windpipes.

What About Dental Surgery and Asthma?

People who have anything more than occasional, mild asthma attacks should not have general anesthetics, such as nitrous oxide (commonly known as laughing gas), at the dentist's office. There is always the possibility of asthma occurring with any general anesthetic, and should it become severe, the dentist may not be able to control it well. Local anesthetics or intravenous sedatives are fine for use at the dentist's office.

If general anesthesia is necessary for dental surgery, it's best to have the surgery performed in a hospital setting.

o o o

Although anesthesia and surgery can present potential problems for the asthmatic, these problems can be avoided if you and your asthma doctor, anesthesiologist, and surgeon have open communication; if you and your doctors properly plan and prepare for your surgery and any asthma complications; and if you and your doctors make attentive efforts to control possible respiratory system complications after surgery.

10

Pregnancy and Asthma

Sally, a 27-year-old asthmatic, was pregnant. During the first 3 months of her pregnancy, she wasn't bothered by the severe asthma that had plagued her several times before she became pregnant. Her symptoms came and went and were fairly mild—occasional chest tightness and shortness of breath. She was relieved that these symptoms subsided without the use of her regular asthma medications since she was afraid to use them for fear they might harm her baby.

At about her fifth month, her symptoms came, but this time they stayed and then worsened over a period of several days. She checked with her doctor, who told her to begin taking her regular asthma medications, which, he assured her, would be safe. Because of her fear that the drugs would hurt her developing baby, she waited longer, but she only got worse. Finally Sally began her asthma medication, but by this time her asthma had a stronghold and didn't respond. She had waited too long to start her medicine and her symptoms snowballed out of control. She needed intensive treatment.

Sally was hospitalized. Because her condition was so severe, she was put on an artificial respirator for several days. Along with this breathing support system, she was given large doses of theophylline, beta stimulators, and steroids. Her doctor was careful to keep her blood oxygen level, which gets dangerously low during a severe asthma attack, up at all times by giving her extra oxygen. Sally responded to this intensive treatment and her asthma attack finally abated. However, she still worried about the treatment's effect on her unborn baby. Her doctor assured her that since her blood oxygen level never got dangerously low, her developing child would probably not have been harmed. He said that not treating her severe condition would have been more harmful to her and the baby than any asthma drug.

Fortunately for Sally, she pulled through and later delivered a healthy, normal baby. But she learned an important lesson—that starting her medication at the first sign of her worsening symptoms could have averted her asthma from getting out of control and requiring intense medication. The next time she would take the necessary measures before her asthma got out of control to ensure her own health safety and the safety of her unborn child.

Asthma is not an uncommon medical problem during pregnancy. In fact, asthma is a major complication in an estimated one percent of all pregnancies. Uncontrolled asthma episodes during pregnancy have been associated with an increase in other problems for both mother and baby. In 15 to 20 percent of all pregnancies with asthma, the asthma is severe enough to require hospitalization, making it a common medical management problem for both the mother-to-be and her doctor.

During pregnancy, the severity of asthma usually stays the same in 41 percent of asthmatics, improves in 36 percent, and worsens in 23 percent. Asthmatics who stay the same or improve during pregnancy usually come from the mild-to-moderate group of asthmatics, whereas asthmatics who worsen during pregnancy are usually severe asthmatics prior to pregnancy. If asthma worsens during a women's first pregnancy, it will usually follow this same pattern in subsequent pregnancies.

Statistics aside, being pregnant and having asthma do not have to result in a worrisome situation. The key to a worry-free pregnancy with asthma can be found in one word—control. For pregnant asthmatic women, control can be achieved through proper medical management with the goals of therapy being identical to those for nonpregnant asthmatics. These goals include the prevention of disabling asthma symptoms, emergency room visits, status asthmaticus (asthma out of control), and respiratory failure. These goals can be easily accomplished, resulting in a smooth, uncomplicated pregnancy with a healthy outcome for both mother and baby.

A management program for the asthmatic mother-to-be must take into account such factors as the physiologic and immunologic changes occurring during pregnancy, the effects of pregnancy on asthma, the effects of asthma on the fetus and mother, and the safe and effective use of drugs for treating asthma during pregnancy. We will address each of these factors in this chapter. In addition, we will discuss breast feeding and asthma drugs as well as breast feeding's possible role in preventing allergy in infants.

What Normal Body Changes Occur During Pregnancy and What Are Their Effects on Asthma?

Pregnancy is associated with many physiologic changes. These normal physiologic changes are caused by multiple hormones, which are mainly produced by the placenta. These hormones promote the growth and development of the fetus and prevent the immunologic rejection of the fetus by the mother. However, they may also affect certain illnesses—such as asthma—in both positive and negative ways. For example, a benefit to the asthmatic can be higher progesterone levels, which may induce relaxation of the windpipes. Of detriment to the asthmatic can be increased levels of progesterone, which may stimulate an increase in the amount of air taken in by each breath. This so-called "hyperventilation of pregnancy" may contribute to a feeling of dyspnea (shortness of breath) and may make a pregnant asthmatic feel as though her asthma is getting worse when, in fact, it is not. In addition, another hormonal change, increased levels of corticosteroids, is considered by some experts to be of some benefit since it decreases the asthmatic response.

Immunologic changes also occur during pregnancy, and in the past were thought to affect the course of asthma. However, it is now known that pregnancy has little effect on IgE antibody formation and probably little effect on the course of asthma.

What Are the Effects of Pregnancy on Asthma?

Generally speaking, about one-fourth of the women with asthma improve when pregnant, one-fourth worsen, and one-half remain the same. Women tend to repeat the same asthmatic pattern with each pregnancy.

There are some common complications related to the effect of pregnancy on asthma we should mention. One of these is something known as reflux esophagitis, which results in what is commonly known as heartburn. This occurs as the enlarging uterus puts upward pressure on the stomach, which may increase the reflux (backward flow) of gastric contents into the esophagus. Bronchodilators used to treat asthma may worsen this reflux by relaxing the esophageal sphincter. If refluxed gastric contents are aspirated into the windpipes (which may occur at night when you are lying down), this could induce more asthma. Elevating the head of the bed and using antacids will reduce reflux and thereby may reduce heartburn and may lessen some asthma symptoms.

Another complication that is indirectly related to the effect pregnancy has on asthma is the development of rhinitis (nasal inflammation). Rhinitis, in a sense, may aggravate the discomfort of asthma because it brings the additional discomfort of a stuffy nose. Rhinitis can occur in pregnant women who have had no problems with it in the past. The occurrence is referred to as "vasomotor rhinitis of pregnancy." Congestion of the nasal passage develops by the end of the first 3 months and progresses throughout the pregnancy. Nasal swelling is especially prominent in the last 2 months before term. These nasal changes are probably due to increased levels of estrogen and progesterone. Women who have allergic or vasomotor rhinitis prior to pregnancy may experience a marked increase in symptoms of nasal congestion. This condition is hard to treat, but some women can get relief by taking a safe decongestant, such as pseudephedrine (Sudafed), and by using topical steroid sprays in the nose on a regular basis. Ask your doctor which products are safe for you to use. Sniffing or spraying a salt-water solution (saline) into the nose may also provide some relief.

Another complication of pregnancy on breathing (mentioned earlier) is "hyperventilation of pregnancy," caused by increased levels of progesterone, resulting in an increase in ventilation. This causes a feeling of shortness of breath, and may worsen underlying asthma. Since sedatives that may be helpful in controlling hyperventilation should not be used during pregnancy, breathing-relaxation techniques are a viable option for controlling this problem. (For more information on hyperventilation and breathing techniques, refer to Chapter 15.)

What Are the Effects of Asthma on the Mother and Fetus?

Severe asthmatics who are *poorly controlled* may have premature labor and their infants are associated with a 35 percent lower birth-weight rate, a 12 percent higher neurologic abnormality rate, and a 28 percent higher mortality rate. In addition, these women have a 12 percent higher mortality rate during pregnancy and childbirth. In contrast, mild asthma results in very little risk to the mother and fetus. However, *all* pregnant asthmatics, regardless of the severity of their condition, will have a minimum of fetal and maternal problems and can expect a favorable outcome of their pregnancy if they are properly controlled with medication.

What Are the Effects of Asthma Medications on the Mother and Fetus?

To achieve good control of asthma during pregnancy, it's often necessary to use drugs. For a drug to be labelled "safe for use in pregnancy," it must be determined safe and effective for the mother and not harmful to the fetus. Unfortunately, it is difficult to be 100 percent certain of the safety of any drug because studies to confirm the safety of drugs are hard to perform. The majority of congenital malformations in infants are *not* the result of properly taken prescription medications. When a medication is used during pregnancy and a congenital malformation occurs, this does not necessarily mean the medication caused the malformation—it could have been be a coincidence.

The critical period for the development of drug-induced fetal abnormalities (teratogenic effects) is between the first 3 to 10 weeks of fetal development. After the first 3 months of pregnancy, the fetal organs are generally formed and birth defects are much less likely to occur.

The following list of commonly used asthma and allergy medications includes descriptions of their effects on the mother and fetus:

Theophylline This drug crosses the placenta, but there have been no cases of fetal malformation reported from it. In all studies, it has not been demonstrated to be harmful if used during pregnancy.

Beta Stimulators (Epinephrine, Ephedrine, Isoproterenol, Metaproterenol, Isoetharine, Albuterol [Salbutamol], Terbutaline, Bitolterol) With the exception of ephedrine, safety for use in pregnancy for the rest of these drugs has not definitely been established, although no known adverse effects have ever been demonstrated. Epinephrine, when used during the first 4 months of pregnancy, has been associated with a slight increased risk of congenital abnormalities; however, this association may have been due to other factors (such as severe asthma) and not to epinephrine itself. Therefore, epinephrine should not be contraindicated in treating an acute asthma attack in a pregnant woman.

With asthma, the benefits of beta stimulators usually outweigh the risks. Inhaled beta stimulators are theoretically safer than the oral forms because they result in a smaller systemic dose. In late pregnancy, use of beta stimulators has the potential for delaying the onset of labor; however, this problem doesn't seem to occur with the usual dosage used in treating asthma.

There is an association between terbutaline and transient strokes in pregnant asthmatic women who have migraines. Therefore, these women should avoid this drug.

Cromolyn Although cromolyn has not been completely studied, no adverse effects have been found, so it is not considered harmful.

Steroids Although much has been written about steroid side effects, there's no evidence that they cause adverse effects on the fetus. It's safer for women with severe asthma symptoms to use systemic steroids than run the risk of getting the fetal damage associated with the low blood-oxygen levels caused by severe asthma. The newer inhaled steroids are also considered safe in pregnancy, although the only one that has been completely studied is beclamethasone.

Antihistamines and Decongestants Because of a slight increased risk of birth defects demonstrated in at least one study, it might be best to avoid brompheniramine, diphenhydramine, hydroxyzine, phenylpropanolamine, and phenylephrine. On the other hand, pseudephedrine, chlorpheniramine, and tripelennamine have been demonstrated to be safe. Other antihistamines and decongestants haven't been studied, but no obvious adverse effects on the fetus are apparent.

Antibiotics　Ampicillin and penicillin are considered safe to use by pregnant women. Erythromycin is safe, but erythromycin with the estolate salt (Ilosone) occasionally causes maternal liver toxicity. Tetracycline, sulfonamides, and troleandomycin are *not* safe for use. There is insufficient data for determining the safety of using other antibiotics.

Iodides (An Expectorant Sometimes Combined with a Bronchodilator)　These should be avoided because of their association with congenital goiter and hypothyroidism in the fetus.

Immunotherapy　Immunotherapy (allergy shots) can be carefully continued during pregnancy in women already receiving immunotherapy who appear to be deriving benefits and who are not experiencing systemic reactions. For those on an increasing antigen-dosage schedule, either very conservative progression or no further dosage increases are recommended so that a systemic reaction (which possibly could induce labor) won't occur.

None of the commonly used asthma medications have any effects on the male reproductive system. If the father was taking medication at the time of conception, it wouldn't affect fetal development.

How Is Asthma Generally Managed in Pregnancy?

As stated earlier in this chapter, the goals of asthma therapy for pregnant women are the same as those for nonpregnant women: to control or prevent disabling asthma symptoms, emergency room visits, status asthmaticus (asthma out of control),and respiratory failure. With the accomplishment of these goals, a pregnant woman can expect a smooth, uncomplicated pregnancy with a healthy outcome for both herself and her baby. Maintenance of good breathing in the mother-to-be is essential to prevent low blood oxygen (hypoxemia) from occurring in the fetus. Hypoxemia is more harmful to the fetus than any of the commonly used asthma medications.

Medical therapy and the avoidance of known triggers are the foundations of asthma treatment. Pregnancy is a good time to reinstitute environmental control of asthma triggers. With environmental control, along with immunotherapy for the extrinsic asthmatic, a pregnant woman may need to take less medication to control her asthma. During pregnancy, as in any other time, you and your doctor must weigh the risks of using a medication against the benefits derived from it. If you find out you're pregnant, don't automatically throw away your asthma medications!

Check with your doctor. You might need them to keep your asthma under control. (For more detailed information on asthma drugs and pregnancy, refer to Chapter 7.)

Finally, no smoking during pregnancy is a wise policy because of smoking's adverse effects on asthma and because it generally results in low birth weight, which is associated with birth defects in the infant.

What Are the Baby's Chances of Getting Asthma?

Asthma can be inherited. Although the genetic transmission of asthma is unclear, some generalities can be made. If neither parent has a history of asthma or a family history of asthma, there is only a small chance they will have a child who will develop asthma. If there is a family history of asthma in either parent, but the parents themselves don't have asthma, the odds of asthma developing in the child are about 10 percent. If only one parent had or has asthma, the chances are approximately 33 percent (1 out of 3) that the child will develop asthma. If both parents had or have asthma, the chances are about 66 percent (2 out of 3) that the child will develop asthma. Asthma can develop shortly after birth in the child or it can occur many years later—sometimes even in old age.

What Are the Effects of Asthma Medications on Breast Feeding?

Often mothers wonder about the effects of a particular asthma drug or treatment on breast feeding. Here are some facts:

- Theophylline is secreted in breast milk, but at 75 percent of the blood level in the mother's body, resulting in a very small dose from the milk to the infant. Occasionally, theophylline has been suspected to cause hyperirritability in the infant; if this occurs, try to take theophylline just after nursing time.

- Beta stimulators, antihistamines, and decongestants are secreted in breast milk in trace amounts, so they do not generally cause problems in the infant.

- It is unknown whether cromolyn is secreted in breast milk. If it is present in milk, it would be unlikely to be absorbed from the gastrointestinal tract of the infant. Therefore, it would not be expected to cause any difficulty.

- Steroids appear in breast milk, and can possibly reach concentrations high enough to affect the infant. Women taking steroids for longer than one month should not nurse.

- There appears to be no reason to limit immunotherapy while nursing.

Although it is possible that allergen may be excreted in milk in trace amounts, it won't harm the infant.

Can Breast Feeding Affect an Infant's Potential To Develop Allergy?

Most studies suggest that if a mother breast-feeds her infant for the first 6 months while also avoiding all major allergenic foods (eggs, soy, wheat, milk, and nuts), the onset of allergic disorders, including extrinsic asthma, can be significantly delayed in her child. Whether or not prevention occurs is not known.

Here are some other precautions that may decrease the incidence or delay the development of allergy in an infant:

- During her last 3 months of pregnancy, the mother-to-be should go on a special diet—avoiding milk, eggs, legumes, cottonseed, seafood (especially shellfish), wheat, and citrus fruits. She should continue this diet during breast feeding to prevent the possible transmission of these common food allergens through her milk.

- She should stop breast-feeding at 6 months, and use Nutramegen instead. This is an enzymatically prepared hydrolysate of casein (not a milk product) with additional additives that make it an ideal formula, providing good nutrition. It is hypoallergenic, but its taste leaves something to be desired.

- There should be the least amount of possible inhalant allergens in the infant's nursery by eliminating sources of animal danders, dust, moulds, and feathers.

- There should be a commitment to a no-smoking policy around the infant.

o   o   o

With proper control, pregnancy and asthma can coexist successfully. Learning about the relationship between your body's changes and asthma, the effects of your pregnancy on asthma, the effects of asthma on you and your unborn baby, and the effects of asthma drugs on pregnancy and breast feeding will give you a foundation for understanding the coexistence of pregnancy and asthma. With this foundation, you will be able to determine the safest control measures for you and your baby.

11

Asthma Out of Control— Complications and Death

Jeremy is a 5-year-old boy with a history of severe eczema, allergic rhinitis, and recurrent asthma. He was eagerly awaiting the following weekend's Halloween festivities; he had his costume ready for a special Halloween party and trick-or-treating. Amidst all the activities, Jeremy developed a cold with a sore throat and runny nose, which triggered his asthma. Although the flare-up seemed slight, his parents began his usual asthma medications promptly to avoid any worsening of his condition. But these treatment measures didn't seem to work this time, and Jeremy's symptoms worsened over the next few days. Late Halloween afternoon his condition began to deteriorate quite rapidly. His breathing became more labored, his nostrils began to flare, and his chest retracted as he gasped for air—his asthma was out of control.

Instead of trick-or-treating, a few hours later Jeremy lay cyanotic in a hospital emergency room, where he had been admitted in severe respiratory distress. Laboratory findings suggested respiratory failure. He was treated with a full course of asthma medications, which did not improve his condition. Instead, his respiratory system began to fail. He was placed on an artificial respirator to breathe for him. Later his lungs collapsed from air leaking into the space around them (this is called pneumothorax—a serious complication of status asthmaticus). This required insertion of chest tubes to remove the air and to allow the lungs to expand again. With continued artificial respiration support, intensive care, and aggressive medical treatment, over the next several days Jeremy improved. He began to move air easier, and was able to tolerate periods of time off the respirator. After another day or two, he was able to be taken off the respirator completely and the chest tubes could be removed without his lungs collapsing.

After his two-week-long nightmare, he left the hospital in good condition. But neither Jeremy nor his parents would ever forget the sequence of events that began as just another asthma flare-up and ended up a life-threatening situation, in which he teetered on the brink of death.

This true story is a good illustration of the severity and danger of status asthmaticus, or asthma that gets so far out of control that it requires hospitalization for treatment. Clinically speaking, status asthmaticus is an acute, severe exacerbation of asthma initially unresponsive to commonly used asthma drugs. Status asthmaticus is considered a life-threatening medical emergency, which is associated with a 1 to 3 percent mortality rate. Its precipitating triggers are the same as those that may provoke any attack of asthma—including exposure to allergens or irritating substances, changes in weather, heavy air pollution, viral infections, or emotional stress. Its major characteristics seem to be widespread narrowing of the airways, heavy mucous secretions, and mucous plugging of the narrowed bronchial tubes.

In the United States, acute asthma attacks account for nearly one million emergency room visits per year with approximately 130,000 hospital admissions per year. In addition to this, each year there are also innumerable emergency visits to physicians' offices for treatment. Asthmatics admitted to the hospital with acute attacks can come from any age group, and any asthmatic can conceivably develop status asthmaticus. No asthmatic—even one considered mild or moderate—is absolutely immune to the development of status asthmaticus. Bearing this in mind, the ability to recognize status asthmaticus and know when to obtain emergency medical treatment for it is very important for anyone who has asthma. Knowing what measures to take if your condition approaches an acute, severe state could save your life!

Status asthmaticus can result in death; consider these startling statistics:

- In 1960 deaths from severe asthma attacks were reported to be 3 per 100,000 people per year; by 1980 this figure had fallen to 1 per 100,000. However, since 1980 the overall death rate has increased to 1.6 per 100,000 people per year.
- Every year there are approximately 5,000 documented deaths resulting from asthma.
- There are 1.5 deaths per every 1,000 active asthma cases every year.
- The mortality rate for hospitalized asthmatics has been reported at 1 to 3 percent.

Fortunately, evidence shows that the mortality rate from asthma could be reduced if physicians, hospital staffs, and asthmatics themselves had a better understanding of asthma and the measures used to control and treat it.

What Factors Could Lead to Status Asthmaticus?

Several factors may lead to the development of an acute, severe attack. They include:

Respiratory infections   Usually viral respiratory-tract infections—such as colds and flu—sensitize the airways so that they are more reactive to triggers, and this results in conditions that are favorable for a worsened state of asthma.

Reactions to inhaled allergens   In some places and at certain times of the year, inhaled allergens exist in such high concentrations that they can lead to status asthmaticus.

Reactions to certain drugs and chemicals   Severe asthma may occur after ingesting aspirin, nonsteroidal anti-inflammatory drugs, and sulfites (to name a few), if you are sensitive to them.

Failure to treat early asthma symptoms with medication   Sometimes asthmatics do not recognize the potential severity of an attack or, for some reason, do not take their prescribed asthma medication in a timely manner. Unfortunately, a lack of proper medication at strategic times can increase chances of developing status asthmaticus.

Undermedication with proper drugs because of unwanted side effects
Admittedly, moderate side effects may occur with therapeutic doses of proper asthma medications; however, undermedication results in improper treatment and can set the stage for an acute attack.

Inadequate use of steroids   Sometimes steroids are not started soon enough after other medications fail, so they do not have time to work. At other times, the steroid dose may be inadequate to control a progressively worsening attack. Or steroids may be stopped too soon from a previous asthma attack, thereby leaving the asthmatic more vulnerable to additional triggers of asthma.

Overuse of nebulized beta-stimulator drugs   If too much inhaled beta-stimulator drug is used, it may actually worsen rather than relieve asthma. Too much inhaled beta stimulator also may have an adverse effect on the heart. (The overuse of a concentrated beta stimulator in hand-held nebulizers was attributed to an epidemic of sudden deaths from asthma in Great Britain in the mid-1960s. During this time the incidence of death from asthma increased fourfold over that in the United States, mainly because the United States did not license the sale of this concentrated product.)

Metabolic acidosis This is the build-up of acid in the bloodstream, caused from other conditions, such as diabetes or kidney failure. It may prevent usual asthma medications from having their desired effect, which could result in status asthmaticus.

Acute emotional stress Emotional stress appears to be able to worsen an already significant asthma condition and may, on occasion, be a major factor in the development of status asthmaticus.

These are just some of the factors that can contribute to the development of status asthmaticus. Be on the lookout for these factors and others you might observe that may lead to asthma out of control. This could help you and your doctor prevent its occurrence in the future.

What Indicators Signify That Asthma Is Getting out of Control?

There are some indicators that can point to an asthma attack getting out of control. These indicators usually warrant your doctor's attention. They include:

- The inability to control asthma symptoms with usual medications over a period of 3 to 4 days. Initially in an asthma attack, airway obstruction is due to airway spasm, which responds well to medication. Later in the attack, obstruction is due to mucous plugging and mucous-membrane swelling, which do not respond well to medication. If your symptoms do not readily respond to asthma medication, the asthma attack is probably progressing to a more severe stage.

- An abrupt, acute onset of more than usual asthma symptoms over a period of hours. This suggests a rapidly deteriorating asthma attack that is out of control.

- Feeling the need to take medication more frequently than prescribed to feel relief (for instance, needing your inhaler every 2 hours instead of every 4 to 6 hours). This suggests that the attack is resistant to usual medication and is out of control.

- The inability to clear mucous secretions by coughing. This suggests that mucus may be plugging your airways, making your asthma more serious and out of control.

If you suspect your asthma may be out of control, contact your physician or go to the emergency room for additional treatment. This may prevent the development of full-blown status asthmaticus and the need for hospitalization.

How Does the Doctor Decide To Hospitalize an Asthmatic?

A doctor looks for certain physical signs in an asthmatic that indicate a severe attack requiring hospitalization. These signs are:

Breath sounds   The doctor observes the intensity of breath sounds and the intensity, location, and timing of wheezes to gain an impression of the severity of the asthma attack. Loud wheezing does not necessarily indicate severe asthma; in fact, sometimes wheezing decreases when asthma worsens because there's less air moving in and out of the lungs. This is especially true when decreased wheezing is associated with increasing shortness of breath.

Chest movements   The physician looks for abnormal chest movements coupled with an increased respiratory rate. During breathing, abnormal chest movements—such as retractions between rib spaces and retraction of the sternum (breastbone)—use of accessory muscles (neck and upper-chest muscles), and flaring of the nostrils signify severe asthma that may require hospitalization.

Vital signs   A rapid pulse and respiratory rate suggest a severe asthma attack. When asthma becomes severe, there may be a fall in the systolic blood pressure and a disappearance of a palpable pulse during inhalation. This is known as pulsus paradoxus—a sign of a severe asthma attack.

Presence of cyanosis   Cyanosis is a bluish discoloration of the lips and nails that occurs when the blood oxygen level is dangerously low; this is an indicator of a severe asthma attack.

Weakness   Weakness or fatigue indicates that an asthmatic is tiring out and not able to continue breathing adequately, which may result in respiratory failure.

Mental function   Development of agitation or disorientation suggests a low blood-oxygen level and/or an increased blood-carbon-dioxide level, which signals severe asthma and respiratory failure.

Presence of some or all of these physical findings usually justifies hospitalization.

Often your doctor will want to objectively measure the severity of an asthma attack by measuring your lung capacity with a pulmonary function test. This simple breathing test can be performed in the doctor's office or an emergency room, and helps determine the need for hospitalization.

Generally, if the measurement of your lung capacity is less than 50 percent of its normal capacity *after* you've taken rapid-acting bronchodilating medications, then hospitalization is usually necessary.

What Typical Experiences Can an Asthmatic Expect in the Hospital?

After admission, the physician will assess the asthmatic to determine the severity of his asthma on a clinical basis (this may have already been done in the physician's office or the emergency room). Assessment consists of a physical examination with emphasis on the major physical findings discussed previously. The doctor will always order lab tests to confirm the physical findings, measure the severity of the asthma, monitor for complications of the asthma, and guide him in the general management of the asthma. Lab tests may include:

- A sputum exam for bacteria and eosinophils (a type of white blood cell that accumulates in the mucus of asthmatics);
- a CBC (complete blood count), including a white cell count that will likely increase from the stress of asthma or complicating infections;
- serum electrolytes to help the doctor determine the fluid and electrolyte needs for intravenous solutions;
- serum theophylline levels to determine if adequate doses of theophylline drugs were being taken before admission to determine the proper dose of intravenous aminophylline or theophylline to be administered in the hospital;
- a chest X-ray to determine complications—such as pneumomediastinum (dissection of air from ruptured air sacs into the tissue spaces between the lungs), pneumothorax (dissection of air from ruptured air sacs into the space between the outside edge of the lung and chest wall, resulting in partial collapses of the lung), atelectasis (collapse of segments of lung tissue from mucous plugging of windpipes), and pneumonia (infection of lung tissue, which can complicate severe asthma);
- a pulmonary function test to measure lung capacity, which may be helpful in determining the severity of an asthma attack and useful in determining when respiratory failure might occur from a severe asthma attack; and
- arterial blood gases, which are helpful in determining the severity of the attack, monitoring the attack, and determining the development of respiratory failure. Blood gas has three major components: the pO_2 (which is a measure of the oxygen level in the blood), the pCO_2 (which is a measure of the carbon dioxide level in the blood), and the pH

(which is the measure of the acidity or alkalinity in the blood). Taking all three measurements into account results in a very accurate picture of asthma's severity. Based on the correlation between blood-gas measurements and asthma severity, the physician will make major decisions regarding the treatment of severe asthma. The following table shows how this is done.

Use of Blood-Gas Measurements to Determine Asthma Severity

Severity of Asthma	Oxygen Blood Level (pO_2)	Carbon Dioxide Blood Level (pCO_2)	pH of Blood
1+ (mild)	normal oxygen blood level (80–100 pO_2)	low carbon dioxide blood level (pCO_2 less than 35)	alkaline blood (increased pH greater than 7.45)
2+ (moderate)	mild decrease in oxygen blood level (60–90 pO_2)	low carbon dioxide blood level (pCO_2 less 35)	alkaline blood (increased pH greater than 7.45)
3+ (severe)	moderate decrease in oxygen blood level (50–60 pO_2)	low carbon dioxide blood level (pCO_2 between 35–45)	alkaline blood pH (between 7.35–7.45)

As asthma becomes more severe, the oxygen blood level (pO_2) falls. In milder (less severe) stages of asthma, the carbon dioxide blood level falls at first because of hyperventilation occurring with the asthma attack, but then changes directions and rises as the attack becomes more severe, leaving the asthmatic tired out and hypoventilating, thus retaining carbon dioxide. When changes in the carbon dioxide blood level occur, the measurement of blood acidity and alkalinity (pH) changes with it.

Carbon dioxide is naturally acidic and when it is "blown off" (by hyperventilating) during the milder stages of asthma, the pH of the blood measures alkaline; when carbon dioxide is retained during the severe stages of asthma, the pH of the blood measures acidic.

Treatment will start as soon as possible after admission. Because asthma is out of control, aggressive treatment will be necessary. Intravenous aminophylline or theophylline, the cornerstone of treatment in status asthmaticus, will be used. If the asthmatic hasn't taken theophylline prior to admission, he usually is given a "loading dose" of 7 milligrams per kilogram of body weight intravenously over 10 to 15 minutes. This is usually followed by a continuous intravenous drip of aminophylline at a dose of 15 to 25 milligrams per kilogram of body weight for 24 hours. Blood theophylline levels are often monitored to help regulate the dose.

Beta stimulators are used in addition to theophylline. Some doctors find repeated doses of epinephrine helpful very early in the attack. However, epinephrine, in some instances, can cause bronchoconstriction rather than bronchodilatation in severe asthma. Consequently, other beta stimulators—which can be given by mouth, injection, or nebulization— are often preferred. Nebulization of beta stimulators is more commonly used for severe asthma. Common drugs for nebulization treatment are isoproterenol, metaproterenol, isoetharine and albuterol (salbutamol). (For more information on the various beta-stimulator drugs used in treating status asthmaticus, refer to Chapter 7.)

Systemic steroids are usually necessary for the treatment of status asthmaticus. Since the effects of steroids take place several hours after they are taken, most doctors will use them early and give them intravenously for quickest action. The most common steroid used in intravenous treatment of asthma is methylprednisolone, which is roughly equivalent in strength and dose to prednisone. The dose for status asthmaticus is 1 milligram for every kilogram of body weight every 4 hours to start and then is rapidly tapered as the asthma improves. With the high doses of steroids used in treating status asthmaticus, the asthmatic's serum potassium may go down and his glucose may go up. This is because high doses of steroids can cause loss of potassium from the kidney and can increase the production of glucose from the liver. These abnormalities of blood chemistry must be corrected if they become severe. Other side effects from short-term high doses of steroids in status asthmaticus are rare to nonexistent.

Besides these asthma medications, antibiotics may be needed to treat complicating pneumonia or sinusitis.

Frequently, the doctor will give extra fluids intravenously to ensure adequate hydration. Adequate hydration reduces the danger of mucus plugging the airways and of falling blood pressure resulting from loss of body fluid, both of which may occur in status asthmaticus.

Oxygen is often necessary to keep the blood level of oxygen in a safe range. Too much oxygen can, on rare occasions, suppress breathing. Therefore, the oxygen level of blood may need to be monitored.

Although most patients with status asthmaticus respond to proper medical treatment, a few do not and progress into total failure of the respiratory system. In these instances, the patients must be given respiratory system support to "buy time" to allow the medical treatment to work. This can be accomplished by the use of an artificial ventilator. However, a life-support system is usually necessary only with very severe asthma.

When patients require artificial ventilation, it usually means their asthma has reached a life-threatening stage due to failure of the respiratory system. Other dangerous complications that can occur with status asthmaticus are:

- cardiac arrhythmias and sudden cardiac arrest,
- shock due to a large drop in blood pressure,
- pneumomediastinum (air in the space between the lungs, due to leakage out of the lungs),
- pneumothorax (air between the chest wall and the lungs, causing the lungs to partially collapse), and
- atelectasis (collapse of the lungs because of mucus plugging the airways).

The complications just listed can and must be controlled or reversed with aggressive treatment. These complications along with respiratory failure are the usual direct cause for death in status asthmaticus.

What Is the Mortality Rate from Asthma?

As stated earlier, from 1960 to 1980 the mortality rate from asthma fell from 3 out of every 100,000 of the total population per year to approximately 1 out of every 100,000; however, the mortality rate from asthma is increasing, as a recent report covering 1980 through 1985 stated mortality at 1.6 out of every 100,000 of the total population per year.

Death is more common in severe asthmatics (those having more than six severe attacks per year despite continued medications). The mortality rate in this particular group of asthmatics may approach 1 to 2 percent per year. Based on previous experience with asthmatics in this group who have died from asthma, we now have knowledge that can help determine which asthmatics in this group are at a greater risk of death. Certain characteristics that occur in some of these asthmatics have been demonstrated to point to an increased risk of death from asthma. Sometimes if the asthmatic, the asthmatic's family, and the physician recognize these risks, the asthmatic may be able to change or modify these characteristics so that the risk of death from asthma can be minimized.

These are some characteristics generally associated with asthmatics who die from asthma:

- not complying with the use of medications required to control asthma because of misunderstanding the need for medicine, choosing to avoid possible side effects or uncomfortable effects of medicine, or failing to appreciate the severity of an asthma attack and thereby delaying taking proper medication;

- only using nonmedical treatment for asthma—such as acupuncture, homeopathic medicines, chiropractic manipulations, and relaxation techniques—to control asthma;

- poor attention to general health care in relationship to asthma (not avoiding known asthma triggers or not observing proper diet and exercise needs);

- presence of multiple emotional problems—such as symptoms of depression, poor self-image, sleep disturbance, appetite problems, excessive anxiety, and behavioral disorders including manipulative use of asthma;

- the presence of multiple social problems—including parental emotional problems, intense marital conflicts, substance abuse, and financial difficulties; and

- disregard of symptoms manifested by an unwillingness to share the presence of symptoms with family or physician, resulting in asthma attacks getting very severe before starting treatment.

Many of these characteristics can be modified or corrected. This would result in a decrease in the incidence of death from asthma and, in general, better control of asthma.

Some other factors that also can point to an increased risk of death from an asthma attack are:

- inadequate steroid dose. Using no steroids or too low of a dose because of undue fear of side effects by the asthmatic, the asthmatic's parents, and occasionally by the physician can result in severe asthma. Sometimes these same side-effect concerns lead to a too rapid discontinuation of steroids from a previous severe attack, resulting in the occurrence of another severe attack soon following;

- time of day of the asthma attack. More deaths occur from an attack between 6 PM and 6 AM because asthma gets worse during this time period and because during this time period there is often a delay in seeking adequate treatment;

- presence of early morning asthma symptoms (3 to 7 AM). This has been associated with sudden, unexpected respiratory arrest and death in asthmatics. Myriad possible reasons for this exist, but their explanations are outside the scope of this book. Suffice it to say that if an asthmatic has early morning symptoms (3 to 7 AM), aggressive medical treatment (using long-acting theophylline drugs at bedtime or a hand-held nebulizer at night) is in order;
- history of seizures associated with asthma attacks. This suggests that the asthma attacks have the potential to become very severe. Seizures are generally due to low blood-oxygen levels occurring with severe asthma;
- age of the asthmatic. Risk of death is greater in asthmatics less than 5 years of age and in the elderly because the treatment itself is more difficult for people in these age groups and complications of asthma leading to death are relatively more common; and
- severe status asthmaticus and asthma that is hard to control on a chronic basis. These conditions are more likely to result in death. With hard to control asthma, the asthmatic, the asthmatic's family, and the physician should try to monitor the condition closely, treat the condition aggressively, and modify the risk factors contributing to asthma getting out of control.

o   o   o

Anyone with asthma should be aware of the signs, symptoms, and contributing factors associated with the development of status asthmaticus. With awareness and prudent action, you can avail yourself of the proper medical measures for preventing and treating status asthmaticus that are so important in guarding against its severe consequences.

Living with Asthma

12
Asthma at School

Asthma, the most chronic disease in childhood, is a condition that must be addressed by schools in their effort to provide an educational program that facilitates effective learning for all students. Three million children under 15 years of age in the United States have asthma, and children with asthma have an approximately 40 percent higher rate of absenteeism from school than nonasthmatic children. Asthma accounts for a staggering 20 percent of all school days lost in elementary and secondary schools. Since, next to home, school is one of the most important environments for children, schools must make a conscientious effort to understand the condition and its impact on the child's education. Furthermore, schools must be willing to take the necessary measures to meet the needs of the asthmatic.

Asthma at school can present some special problems, not only for asthmatics but for the educators who work with them. Numerous problems can exist through misunderstanding or lack of knowledge about asthma and the asthmatic. Even when school personnel have a firm understanding of asthma, it may still be difficult for them to know what to do in certain situations and how to go about helping the asthmatic cope at school. Nonetheless, coping with asthma is not an unrealistic goal in the school setting.

To effectively cope with asthma at school, everyone involved—the child, parent, physician, and all major school personnel—must make a collective commitment to recognize, understand, and take action in order to prevent or control asthma at school. This commitment should be undertaken in a positive spirit with the purpose of best meeting the emotional, physical, and academic needs of the child. Sounds difficult, doesn't it? Regardless, it can be accomplished through the three measures mentioned earlier: recognizing asthma (realizing it exists); understanding the causes, triggers, and consequences of asthma; and acting upon the information to help the asthmatic child have a positive and healthy educational experience. Remember, achieving these measures requires a commitment from everyone involved. Read on to see how to go about making these ideas become realities.

Recognition

Obviously, the parents and child need to recognize that asthma exists in the youngster—this goes without saying! But it's also important for the parents to make the school personnel aware of their child's asthma. If your child has asthma, request a meeting with the principal, teacher, and school nurse at the beginning of the school year. Be prepared to inform them:

- that your child has asthma, and tell them what asthma is;
- that you wish to work collectively to help your child feel comfortable and free to function at school;
- about the causes and triggers of asthma, and the treatment measures your child will need at school to cope with asthma; and
- that there are ways in which they can go about helping your child cope with asthma at school (there is more on this point later).

Communicating this important information to school personnel involved with your child is the foundation for the work you will do together.

Understanding and Action

After the condition has been addressed and recognized, a better and more thorough understanding of asthma and the problems it can create for the child at school needs to begin. We've compiled a list of several problems faced by the asthmatic at school. In addition to the problems, we've supplied a few suggestions on how they can be handled. Use this list as a starting place; show it to the school personnel when you address the issue of your child's asthma. You've probably already thought of some of these problems yourself. If you haven't considered approaching the school personnel with a list such as this, please do so. By presenting these items and discussing them with your child's educators, you will be stepping beyond mere recognition of your child's condition and moving towards *action* in helping school personnel and your child better cope with asthma at school.

Common Problems Faced by the Asthmatic at School

Absenteeism   Even with proper control measures at home, asthmatics tend to miss school more frequently than nonasthmatics (remember those staggering statistics!). Sometimes parents are afraid to let their child go to school with a particularly bad bout of asthma because they feel better keeping an eye on the symptoms at home. Often schools don't understand that asthma isn't contagious, so a child who continually coughs and wheezes may be viewed as someone who needs to stay home and not be around classmates. Although both of these theories are wrapped in good intentions, they don't keep the child in the classroom where he belongs to achieve the total learning experience.

Solutions: Absenteeism can be minimized by optimal medical control of asthma, better understanding of asthma through open communication between parents and school personnel, and by the school providing ready access to tutoring sessions (before and after school or in the child's home) to help keep asthmatic children abreast of the learning experience.

It's sometimes difficult for parents to decide whether to keep their asthmatic child at home or send him to school. The following guidelines, established by the International Center for Interdisciplinary Research on Immunologic Diseases at Georgetown University in Washington, D.C. (which we have modified), should be helpful.

Keep your child at home if he has:

- evidence of infection, sore throat, earache, painful neck glands, fatigue, and headache;
- fever over 100 °F orally;
- wheezing and/or coughing associated with labored breathing one hour after taking medication;
- weakness or tiredness that makes it hard to participate in usual daily activities; and
- persistent shortness of breath, even after taking medicine.

Send your child to school, even if he has:

- stuffy nose but no wheezing;
- wheezing and coughing that clear after taking medicine;
- minor asthma symptoms, while still having the ability to carry out usual daily activities;
- wheezing and coughing that are mild but still persist after taking medicine (as long as there is good communication between the school personnel and parents), asthma medications are available at school, and the parents can be easily reached.

Another kind of absenteeism problem can exist if an asthmatic uses his illness as an excuse for not participating in the classroom situation. Parents and teachers should encourage the child to be honest and help him learn to cope so that he can be a part of the class. Sometimes the firm approach here is best.

Peer-Group Pressure   Generally, classmates do not understand asthma and its symptoms, so they regard the asthmatic as "different" or even "sickly." Because of this, the asthmatic can be subject to ridicule by his classmates. Such a situation creates feelings of not belonging and inferiority in the asthmatic. Indeed, nonacceptance by peers can reinforce any negative feelings of being "different" that already exist in the asthmatic.

Solutions: It is best to minimize this problem by efforts to educate classroom students about common diseases and their symptoms. Stressing that each person in the room is unique sets a positive tone for fostering understanding among classmates. Taking the asthmatic aside and giving gentle reassurance helps, too.

Taking Medicines at School Asthmatics often don't take their medicines at school because they want to hide the fact that they need medication. On the other hand, some school policies make it difficult for the willing student to take medicines in a timely fashion at school. Children should not have to worry about finding the school nurse or secretary to dispense their medications if they are old enough to take on this responsibility themselves. Sometimes asthmatics need to take medications immediately upon development of symptoms and therefore need medicine at hand. Also, leaving the classroom and going to the office to get the medicine can draw unwanted attention to themselves.

Solutions: Asthmatics who are treated positively at school will probably have a better feeling about taking medicines when they're at school; once again, classroom education is the key.

If a child needs an inhaler immediately to avert an attack, then he should be able to carry it with him at all times. Schools need to deal individually with the asthmatic's needs, and they need to make workable arrangements for timely dispensing of medication. For some schools, this might require a reevaluation of their present policies concerning medication.

Side Effects from Medication Unfortunately, some asthma medications have unwanted, yet common, side effects. Irritability and drowsiness, the side effects from some medications, can affect a child's conduct and learning ability. Also, sometimes a child's attention span dwindles after taking medication. Add these side effects to an inability to concentrate because of a poor night's sleep (due to an asthma attack) and there's bound to be some learning problems.

Solutions: For side effects, such as irritability and drowsiness, communication between the parents and the teacher is the key. Teachers should realize that changes in behavior may be due to asthma medicines and should communicate behavior changes to the parents (the parents and doctor may not be aware that these behavior changes are occurring). In some instances a change in medicine or a modification of the dose may be possible.

To get around the problem of the short attention span, a teacher could have the student work on short attention-span activities related to specific skills to help the child cope and still keep up with the class.

General Classroom Problems These behavioral problems in the class-room are commonly associated with asthmatics:
- passive behavior and fear of participating in activities;
- poor peer interaction;
- fear of tackling new learning material;
- denial of the illness (which could lead to a severe attack from lack of proper treatment); and
- depression, anxiety, or embarassment because of appearance problems related to asthma—such as barrel chest, eczema, and height or weight problems.

Solutions: It is best to look at general classroom behavior problems in light of the individual asthmatic. If the child exhibits any of the problems in the preceding list to the degree that impairs his total functioning in the classroom, the teacher should suggest counselling to help the child cope, and again, communication between the parents and the teacher is the key. Make certain to notify other school personnel of these problems, too.

Participating in Physical Education Class Physical education class presents specific problems for those asthmatics whose asthma is triggered by exercise. Unfortunately, some instructors do not know about exercise-induced asthma (EIA), and may think a student is trying to get out of participating by saying he can't breathe. On occasion an asthmatic may be unknowingly pushed beyond his capacity because of an instructor's lack of understanding of exercise-induced asthma. On the other hand, a student may be embarrassed to reveal his asthma problem to the teacher and may push himself beyond his physical capacity.

Solutions: Make the teacher aware of the various asthma triggers— especially extrinsic triggers, such as running activities, and environmental triggers, such as cold, dry air and allergic seasons of the year. Encourage your child to tell the teacher when he is having problems with asthma and needs to refrain from physical education activities. Ask your doctor to supply a letter to the instructor stating the triggers of your child's asthma and how these triggers affect his physical performance (you can show your doctor the sample letter that follows to use as a guide).

Sample Letter to School

Date: _____

_____ is presently under my care for asthma. Frequent exercise will cause asthma. _____ should be excused from all physical activity that causes asthma. This will vary from day to day, and _____ must be trusted to decide for himself if a particular activity on a given day is too much. Physical exercise is good for an asthmatic, but only to the extent that the individual asthmatic can tolerate on a given day.

Sincerely,

Physician's name

The teacher should trust the asthmatic to know his own limits. The parents and teacher should encourage the asthmatic to look at his physical abilities in view of asthma in an honest, fair, and realistic manner. They should also encourage him to never exaggerate or downplay his condition. Asthmatics can take a certain medication *before* physical education class to avert their symptoms—check with your doctor about a prescription. (For more information about sports and asthma, refer to Chapter 13.)

Recess Children love recess, but this carefree time can precipitate an attack for many asthmatics. Physical activity and breathing cold, dry air are major asthmatic triggers. Couple this with the allergic season and asthmatic children can be in real trouble! But often asthmatic children want to go outdoors for fun and to interact with their peers regardless of symptom consequences.

Solutions: It's a good idea for parents of asthmatics to alert school personnel that breathing cold, dry air and doing exercise are asthma triggers and that certain seasons of the year may be worse than others. Parents should send a note to the school requesting that their child be allowed to stay indoors during recess on certain days when going outside may trigger asthma (sending a note is a good reminder for everyone!).

The parents and teacher should educate the child to recognize asthma triggers so that he will realize that missing recess may be important to his health on certain days of the year.

Perhaps the teacher could let the child do something he enjoys while the rest of the class is outdoors—such as helping do chores around the classroom, doing artwork, reading, or listening to music.

Classroom Allergens Allergens abound in a classroom! Mould spores, animal dander from classroom pets, and dust can be constant triggers to a susceptible asthmatic.

Solutions: Furry pets could be replaced with fish; also, increased dust-minimization and mould-reduction measures on the part of the custodial staff would be very helpful. Although allergens can't realistically be wiped out, they can be minimized with effort.

Hearing Loss Nasal problems associated with asthma may cause intermittent hearing problems for children. Teachers should be on the lookout for the asthmatic who has trouble following verbal directions; he could have a temporary hearing problem, resulting from nasal congestion blocking his eustachian tubes.

Solutions: Children with suspected hearing loss should be assessed for possible ear ventilation tubes to help their hearing. Children can take medication to counteract the congestion and improve their hearing, too.

Emergency Situations The asthmatic may develop a severe attack at school and need immediate medical assistance.

Solutions: Parents and school personnel should talk about what to do in an emergency situation *before* it occurs. The child needs to know how to tell when he's in trouble and the school staff need to know what measures to take to help the child while the parents are being notified. Proper planning will minimize the stress of an emergency situation, and may even save the child's life.

Special Diet Occasionally an asthmatic must avoid certain foods. This can present problems if the youngster wants to eat the cafeteria lunch with friends.

Solutions: The cafeteria staff could be alerted to the child's needs, and help him in making certain selections. Or the child could take his lunch regularly and only eat cafeteria food on days when the menu won't trigger asthma (most schools provide the month's cafeteria menu to parents; if yours doesn't, ask for one).

Guidelines for Working Together

A collective commitment on the part of the child, parents, physician, and school personnel can help the asthmatic child have a rewarding educational experience. To help each member best fulfill his part, here are some suggestions and guidelines (use this as a checklist).

The asthmatic child needs to:
- understand the condition and know when his body is signalling asthma;
- know his asthma medicines—their names, when to take them, how they help him, and possible side effects he may experience when taking them;
- know who to tell and what to do when asthma flares;
- know his limitations;
- regard his teachers as friends who are interested in him and his asthma and who want to help him;
- never exaggerate asthma symptoms to avoid physical activities or participation in the classroom; and
- never downplay his asthma.

The parents need to:
- recognize asthma symptoms, seek medical diagnosis, and understand their child's condition;
- understand their child's medications and their common side effects, help their child learn about his medications, and make sure the medications are taken properly;
- discuss with their child his capabilities and limitations, and trust him to know those limitations;
- communicate their child's condition, triggers, medicines, capabilities, and limitations to proper school personnel;
- keep lines of communication open with their child to facilitate understanding and positive feelings; and
- calmly reassure their child concerning asthma, present a positive "can-do" attitude about coping with asthma, and provide emotional support.

The physician needs to:

- diagnose asthma and establish a treatment program that includes medical and preventive measures;
- discuss the condition thoroughly with the child and parent, stressing those triggers that could exacerbate asthma in a school setting;
- be willing to discuss the child's condition with school personnel, if needed; and
- provide the school with information about the condition and its limitations (using a note, such as the sample letter for the physical education class).

School personnel need to:

- recognize asthma symptoms and understand the condition, and realize that asthma can affect a child's school experience and that his school experience can affect his asthma;
- be supportive of programs that take into consideration the needs of the asthmatic;
- be trusting and flexible in allowing the child to take medicine at school;
- be aware of the children in class who have asthma, and be aware of each child's asthma triggers and limitations (this includes establishing realistic physical education goals);
- become involved with parents and doctors in a team effort to help the child cope with asthma at school;
- help the child avoid common asthma triggers at school;
- encourage the child to take medications, and be aware of common side effects and their impact on classroom performance;
- be observant and aware of the child's changing condition;
- encourage active classroom involvement and participation that is realistic with the child's limitations;
- provide positive encouragement if the child misses school because of asthma;
- trust the asthmatic to know his limitations; and
- avoid labelling the child as "sick"—treating him positively and matter-of-factly instead.

One last point on working together. When a child is quite sick most of the time, he may have to deal with many of the problems we've discussed in this chapter, and this can be overwhelming for both the child and his teachers. In this situation, you may want to consider writing up a "teamwork contract" to help everyone involved live up to the collective commitment. Once the parents, school personnel, and the asthmatic child have had an initial meeting, writing a contract is a good step to take to make sure that everyone understands his responsibilities. From time to time the team should get together to reevaluate how well the terms of the contract are working out and to see what areas people need to work on or revise. This is a good way for everyone to keep a handle on the situation.

We encourage you to write your own personal "teamwork contract." Include every member of the team in the writing process; that way they can feel responsible for their input and involvement in making the team effort work.

o   o   o

The guidelines in this chapter are not the complete answers to the problems inherent in coping with asthma at school, but they are a conscientious, realistic starting point for everyone involved. Teamwork based on accurate information and specific ways to transform that information into action can make coping with asthma at school a reality. Try the suggestions in this chapter; maybe they will work for you.

13

Exercise, Sports, and Asthma

Tim, a 15-year-old high school athlete and sports enthusiast, was a member of his high school track team. He was a promising, dedicated runner. For all his determination, however, some days he just couldn't perform as well as others; he would become easily winded and his chest would hurt. Tim became frustrated at his inconsistent performance. While his physical education teacher recognized Tim's athletic potential, he, too, was bewildered by Tim's inconsistent performance patterns. He mentioned Tim's behavior to his wife, a nurse who worked for an allergist. She thought it sounded as if Tim might have asthma. The teacher conferred with Tim and his parents, who decided to secure a medical opinion. Sure enough, Tim did have asthma—*exercise-induced asthma*. He was given medication to prevent his attacks. With his newfound freedom from symptoms, Tim's athletic prowess flourished, and he went on to become the next year's number one cross-country runner in the state.

The story about Tim is true. For years, exercise-induced asthma experienced by Tim and many others was not understood. Asthma triggered by exercise, although common, wasn't readily recognized, especially if exercise was the only trigger. Sometimes, asthmatics were viewed by others as being malingerers if they weren't able to perform physical activities. This lack of recognition often created confusion and poor self-image problems for asthmatics, and perpetuated a lack of general knowledge about exercise-induced asthma. Medically speaking, we know that many things can trigger asthma. One of these things is exercise. Through awareness of asthma and this exercise trigger, athletes, physical fitness enthusiasts, and people who live and work with these individuals will be in a position to help control and cope with the problems associated with exercise-induced asthma.

Over the last fifteen years much work has been done to determine the cause, mechanisms, treatment, and control of exercise-induced asthma. In part, this work was stimulated by problems Olympic athletes were encountering in coping with their asthma. Many Olympic asthmatic athletes have, in fact, overcome exercise-induced asthma with proper medical treatment that lies within the rules of the International Olympic Committee, and have won medals in at least one of the Olympic games since 1956. Likewise, the performance problems encountered by all athletes can be overcome. In this chapter, we address asthma's relationship to exercise and athletics, and the various ways exercise-induced asthma can be treated and controlled.

What Is Exercise-Induced Asthma?

Exercise-induced asthma, or EIA, is the development of typical asthma symptoms (wheezing, coughing, and shortness of breath), triggered by exercise. It can occur in all asthmatics, but usually occurs more often in children than adults since children are naturally more active. Sometimes, asthma occurs *only* after exercise and at no other times in a person's life, making it difficult to diagnose.

During the first few minutes of exercise, the bronchial tubes normally expand. But then several minutes later, there is an onset of bronchospasm, which usually becomes very significant within 5 to 10 minutes after stopping exercise. Symptoms—such as chest tightness, shortness of breath, wheezing, and coughing—can be mild, moderate, or severe, depending on the individual, the type of exercise, and the various environmental conditions that are present during exercise. The physical exertion must be intense enough to raise the heart rate to 180 beats per minute in children and 150 to 160 beats per minute in adults. In other words, exertion of about 70 percent of a person's aerobic power is most likely to trigger EIA. Symptoms may last up to an hour, then gradually subside. In about one-third of the people with EIA, there is a second, delayed asthmatic reaction that occurs about 4 hours later.

What Causes Exercise-Induced Asthma?

During exercise, rapid breathing brings large volumes of cool, dry air into the bronchial tubes. As the airways work to warm and humidify the incoming air, there is a loss of moisture from the bronchial tubes. This loss of moisture is considered the major cause of EIA, although heat loss may be an additional stimulus. These losses cause the release of potent chemical mediators (known as neutrophil chemotactic factor and histamine), which in turn causes spasms in the windpipes.

What Factors Increase the Chances
of Exercise-Induced Asthma?

A variety of factors that may be present when a person exercises can increase his chances of experiencing exercise-induced asthma. These factors include very cold dry air, allergy-producing substances such as pollen and air pollution, and a viral infection such as a cold or the flu in the person exercising.

Running sports, certain gymnastics, and skiing are the greatest triggers for exercise-induced asthma since they are performed strenuously for long time periods. Cycling is an intermediate trigger, and swimming and walking are lesser triggers. However, these differences may be largely due to the environment in which these exercises are performed. For example, running in a cold, dry environment invites EIA. Swimming, on the other hand, usually occurs in a warm, humid environment, which in itself is protective against exercise-induced asthma.

What Are Some Clues To Look for
in Exercise-Induced Asthma?

If you are involved in sports, or you live or work with an athlete, you can use these clues to tell if exercise-induced asthma might be a problem:

- continuous coughing after physical exertion;
- varied performance in exercise-related activities from day to day and season to season;
- frequent periods of tiring with exercise;
- ability to perform better in the latter half of sports events (see description of refractory period on page 159);
- complaints of chest pain, burning, and/or tightness after exercise;
- wheezing within a few minutes after exercise; and
- frequent problems with nasal congestion from hay fever and colds (a common association with asthma).

How Is Exercise-Induced Asthma Diagnosed?

EIA is not always recognized because people can have it and not know it. But once it is suspected, a thorough medical evaluation is necessary to obtain an accurate diagnosis.

An exercise test performed on a treadmill or an exercise bicycle for 6 to 8 minutes in the physician's office is one way to diagnose exercise-induced asthma and to determine its severity. The amount of exercise performed during the test should increase the heart rate of the individual to at least 90 percent of the predicted maximum for his age. To determine the development of EIA, pulmonary function tests are measured before exercise begins and at 5-minute intervals after exercise stops.

A methacholine challenge test (this is the asthma-provoking test discussed in Chapter 5) can also be performed in the physician's office to diagnose EIA. Because it's simpler to perform, this test is used more often than the exercise test.

With an inexpensive device, called a peak flowmeter, an athletic performance can be monitored in the field under the actual conditions in which athletes perform. Such direct monitoring, done just before and 5 to 10 minutes after an athletic performance, is helpful for adjusting medications and for determining how many precompetitive warm-up sprints may be necessary in preventing an attack.

How Can Exercise-Induced Asthma Be Treated and Controlled?

The best treatment for controlling EIA is medication. The best medicines for the prevention and treatment of EIA are beta-stimulating drugs, which dilate the windpipes. According to studies, the best beta stimulant to use is albuterol (salbutamol). You can prevent an attack by inhaling two puffs of albuterol 15 to 30 minutes before exercise, or by taking 2 to 4 milligrams one hour before exercise. Protection usually lasts 4 hours, but there is partial protection for up to 6 hours. For additional prevention, you can inhale cromolyn sodium, a drug known to inhibit the release of chemical mediators in the lungs, along with the beta stimulant before exercise. Both drugs can be repeated up to six times per day to provide continuous prevention and treatment for EIA.

Theophylline, another kind of drug that dilates the windpipes, isn't as effective as cromolyn or beta stimulants, but it can help in preventing EIA. Theophylline can be taken in a long-acting preparation to keep airways maximally opened around the clock. Theophylline may have an additive effect to beta-stimulating drugs in controlling EIA.

Evidence suggests that the more open the airways are before exercise, the less severe EIA will be. Therefore, it may be good to use bronchodilators—such as theophylline and beta stimulants—and cromolyn on a continuous basis if you are going to be active regularly.

In addition to medication, warm-up sprints are effective in preventing EIA. A series of eight to ten 30-second sprints performed within one hour prior to an athletic event may cause the windpipes to become refractory to the development of EIA during the time of the event. What this means is that further exercise for a period of up to 4 hours will not cause asthma or as much asthma as it ordinarily would if the sprints hadn't been performed.

Also, certain self-help techniques can be used in controlling EIA, especially if you have associated hyperventilation (excessive rapid breathing). Basically, EIA is due to rapid breathing in an asthmatic that causes loss of moisture and possible loss of heat from his airways. Simple hyperventilation without doing any exercise can also cause asthma. Additionally, participants in competitive sports often experience anxiety, which, in itself, can cause hyperventilation and exacerbate asthma. Consequently, knowing self-help techniques to reduce hyperventilation and encourage relaxation can help control EIA.

One such technique is a form of progressive muscle relaxation that is done prior to exercise. Sit or lie in a comfortable position and concentrate on tensing and then relaxing specific muscles in your body to create an awareness of what your body feels like when it is tense and when it is relaxed. This technique is usually done with one muscle group at a time, starting with the lower body muscles and moving up to the muscles of the head and neck. With practice, you will be able to achieve a relaxed state even before an athletic event.

Another relaxation technique is relaxed (diaphragmatic) breathing, also known as belly breathing. Your diaphragm is the large muscle below your rib cage. To breathe with your diaphragm, you need to breathe in slowly through your nose and exhale slowly through pursed lips. Your breathing should also be relaxed. If done correctly, there should be movement of your abdominal muscles and little or no movement of your chest muscles. To check yourself, rest your hand on your abdomen; your hand should rise with your abdomen during inhalation and fall with your abdomen during exhalation if you are breathing with your diaphragm. You should do belly breathing for 5 minutes whenever you feel anxious and are on the verge of overbreathing and hyperventilating before an athletic event. (For more detailed information about progressive muscle relaxation and belly breathing techniques, see Chapter 15.)

It is important to remember that these self-help measures are effective in controlling hyperventilation but not bronchospasm itself. However, since hyperventilation and exercise may contribute towards bronchospasm for the same reason, applying these self-help techniques will help control asthma.

o   o   o

Certainly, exercise-induced asthma can be avoided by eliminating all exercise from a person's life. But, obviously, this would be unrealistic and undesirable. Exercise is an important part of the totality of our lives. To refrain from exercise would be detrimental to the normal physical and emotional development of children, would restrict adults unnecessarily, would foster poor physical fitness, and would have unfavorable effects on cardiovascular function and general health. Instead of eliminating exercise from our lives, it is better to find ways of preventing asthma related to exercise from happening. Then we can live our lives to the fullest potential. With proper medical treatment, exercise warm-ups, and self-help techniques, an asthmatic can successfully perform or even compete in most physical activities.

14

Asthma and the Workplace

Asthma caused from the workplace environment is called *occupational asthma*. For many centuries the hazards of respirable occupational fumes, dusts, and vapors have been recognized. However, over the last two decades, asthma at the workplace has become an increasing problem. This is due to the rapid development and diversity in industry creating many new chemicals and other new substances to which we are exposed. Many of these substances can trigger asthma by either allergic or nonallergic reactions.

Asthma from the workplace is now estimated to account for 2 to 5 percent of adult asthma in Western society and as much as 15 percent of adult asthma in Japan.

The development of asthma at the workplace depends upon the type of substances the worker is exposed to (only certain substances cause asthma), how much of the substance is airborne and inhaled (resulting in significant exposure), and the individual's sensitivity (whether he's allergic or nonallergic) to the substance. Sensitivity can take a while to develop. There is a latent, or sensitizing, period of exposure before asthma develops. This sensitizing period may vary from just a couple of days to many years, but in the majority of occupational asthma cases it is usually a matter of a few months. A multitude of allergens are capable of being offending agents; the list ranges from industrial chemicals to agricultural products.

In most workplace environments associated with occupational asthma, only 5 to 10 percent of the workers exposed to known sensitizers will develop asthma while they're working. Occupational asthma symptoms are no different from regular asthma symptoms—those of wheezing, coughing, and shortness of breath. They often occur just after exposure to the offending agent, but not always. In fact, often these symptoms occur hours after exposure. There are three basic symptom patterns, or reactions, related to occupational asthma:

- immediate reaction, when asthma symptoms develop within minutes after exposure to the offending agent and clear within 1 to 2 hours;

- late reaction, when asthma symptoms develop within 1 to 8 hours after exposure to the offending agent and last from 12 to 36 hours (therefore, these symptoms can occur at night, many hours removed from the workplace); and

- dual reaction, when asthma symptoms occur immediately as well as much later in the same person.

These reactions can result in various asthma patterns that suggest that the asthma is related to the workplace. Look for the following asthma patterns:

Similar amounts of asthmatic symptoms on each workday Symptoms develop during each working time period, but improve rapidly after the asthmatic leaves work and are completely gone before the next workday begins (short recovery time from the asthma).

Progressive worsening of asthma symptoms throughout the working week This occurs because of a longer recovery time from occupational asthma of between 1 to 3 days. Thus, each morning the asthma is worse than the previous morning and worsens further during the day. The asthma improves when the individual is away from the workplace for several days.

Progressive worsening of asthma symptoms week by week This occurs if the asthma recovery time is very prolonged (more than 3 days) so that the asthma is still present even after a weekend away from work.

Maximal asthma symptoms on the first day of the work week Asthma symptoms occur on the first day of the work week but then improve throughout the week. This is the least common asthma pattern, and usually occurs only in occupational asthma of cotton workers (known as byssinosis).

What Makes an Individual Likely To Develop Occupational Asthma?

Atopy (allergy) Individuals susceptible to allergy are more likely to develop occupational asthma, and the condition usually develops sooner than for nonallergic people.

Exposure to high doses of an offending agent A higher dose of an offending agent causes greater sensitivity and/or irritation of the windpipes.

Previous asthma   All asthmatics, whether intrinsic or extrinsic, are at risk of developing asthma symptoms from the workplace since their hyperreactive airways are extra sensitive to irritating fumes and vapors, which abound in many workplace environments. (Since their asthma condition was preexisting, this may not be considered true occupational asthma.)

Length of time exposed to the offending agent   Whether or not a person develops occupational asthma depends on the length of time he is exposed to the offending agent. However, the length of time of exposure before sensitization and subsequent symptoms appear can be as short as a few months or as long as 10 years.

The offending agent   Occupational asthma occurs prevalently in certain occupations more than others and upon exposure to certain agents more than others. This depends on the asthma-triggering potency of the agents.

Why Is It Important To Know if Asthma Is Occupational or Nonoccupational?

In the last few years occupational asthma has attracted much medical attention. A large number of previously unknown occupational causes of asthma have been discovered, particularly in the chemicals, plastics, and electronics industries. However, as we've mentioned, existing asthma *exacerbated by* exposure to occupational irritants is not commonly considered true occupational asthma. In its strictest sense, occupational asthma is asthma *caused by* exposure to inhaled sensitizing agents in the workplace. This distinction is important since occupational asthma is becoming increasingly accepted as a compensable disease.

In Germany and Finland, people can claim individual disablement benefits for occupational asthma. In England, occupational asthma became a prescribed disease in 1982 under the National Injuries Laws, thereby entitling affected individuals to compensation from central government funds. In the United States, occupational asthma is the basis of many individual legal actions and is generating much legislative concern at both state and federal levels. Because of these legal trends, occupational asthma must be distinguished from nonoccupational asthma and recognized as a unique work-related phenomenon.

What Kind of Reactions Are Involved in Occupational Asthma?

Occupational asthma can be caused by both allergic and nonallergic reactions. The allergic reaction that causes occupational asthma is the same as the allergic reaction that causes extrinsic asthma: An IgE antibody made by the asthmatic reacts with the offending agent, causing the release of chemical mediators, which induces asthma. Individuals with sensitivity to common outdoor and indoor allergens are at greater risk of developing occupational asthma when this mechanism is involved.

One nonallergic reaction involves inhaling irritating substances that can trigger an asthma attack. People with both intrinsic and extrinsic asthma who have hypersensitive airways are more sensitive than others to these substances. Another nonallergic reaction is a chemical change in the lungs caused by the offending agent, resulting in asthma.

What Occupational Agents Can Cause Asthma at the Workplace?

We have divided the agents that can cause occupational asthma into the following categories: industrial chemicals; metal salts; drugs and enzymes; insects, animals, and fungi; wood dusts; and grain, plant dust, and vegetable gums. We have also included a special section on byssinosis, a form of occupational asthma caused by exposure to cotton, flax, or hemp dust.

INDUSTRIAL CHEMICALS

Isocyanates   A number of isocyanates are used widely in industry in the production of polyurethanes, plastics, paints and varnishes, elastomers, adhesives, and flexible and rigid foams.

The isocyanate list includes diphenylmethane diisocyanate (MDI), hexamethaline diisocyanate (HDI), naphthylene diisocyanate (NDI), and the most widely used of these compounds, toluene diisocyanate (TDI).

Isocyanates are very common occupational agents; as many as 500,000 workers in the United States come in contact with them in the course of their work experience. Isocyanates have a pungent, acrid odor. They affect the lungs of some people more than others, possibly because of an allergic sensitivity, but other mechanisms may also be involved.

TDI is the most common isocyanate causing occupational asthma. Occupational asthma develops in 5 percent of the workers regularly exposed to it. With regular, consistent exposure, it may take weeks to years for a worker to become sensitized and develop symptoms. Symptoms usually improve when contact with TDI ceases, but this improvement can take days.

The table that follows shows some of the occupations associated with isocyanate agents.

The Most Common Occupations Associated with Isocyanate Agents

Isocyanate agent	Occupations involved
TDI	Flexible foam manufacturing
	Toy making
	Boat building
	Refrigerator manufacturing
	Printing and laminating
	Insulating
	Plastics producing
MDI	Insulating
	Foundry working (plastic moulds)
	Printing
	Rigid foam manufacturing
HDI	Automobile paint spraying
NDI	Synthetic rubber manufacturing
	Foundry working (plastic moulds)

Acid Anhydrides These substances are used widely in the plastics and paint industries as hardening agents for epoxy resins and as raw materials in plasticizers. Composing the list of anhydrides are phthalic anhydride (PA), hexahydrophthalic anhydride (HHDA), tetrachloraphthalic anhydride (TCPA), himic anhydride (HA), and trimellitic anhydride (TMA).

As much as about 20 percent of the workers exposed to anhydrides develop respiratory sensitization. Exposure can occur from dusts, aerosols, fumes, and vapors. The type of exposure depends on the industrial process in which the chemicals are used.

Acid anhydrides induce asthma through both an allergic and irritant reaction in the windpipes. On occasion with exposure to TMA and TCPA, there can be a late asthma reaction (several hours after exposure), occurring with flulike symptoms, such as chills, fever, malaise, and muscle pains. On rare occasions, exposure to high concentrations of TMA fumes can cause a pneumonialike infiltrate in the lungs that occurs with anemia and coughing up blood.

An interesting phenomenon occurs in what is called "meat-wrappers' " asthma. During meat-wrapping, labels containing phthalic anhydride are heated to adhere to the polyvinyl-chloride meat wrapping. In this process, phthalic anhydride fumes are released and can induce asthma.

Colophony Fumes or vapors from fluxes (substances used to promote fusion of metals in soldering and welding) containing colophony (pine-tree resin) can cause occupational asthma. Colophony is heavily used in the electronics industry, where it is a primary ingredient of soldering fluxes. In the process of soldering, fumes are liberated into the breathing zones of workers soldering electronic circuit boards. Colophony fumes also occur from the use of hot melt glue, and are aerosolized when used in deodorants, used as emulsifiers, and used in cutting ores. Although colophony usually induces asthma after being heated, it can induce asthma after exposure at room temperature. Unheated colophony is widely used as an adhesive, surface coater, and varnish, and is sometimes used as an ingredient in printing ink and to increase water resistance in paper. Occasionally, it is used to stop slippage of machine belts, tennis shoes, and other sporting equipment.

Colophony is thought to induce asthma through an allergic reaction, but it also acts as an irritant and induces symptoms in intrinsic asthmatics.

The average period of exposure to colophony at the workplace before asthma develops is 4 years, but sometimes exposure can be as short as one month or as long as 20 years before asthma develops.

Sensitive individuals may even react to disinfectants and cleaning substances commonly used around the home because they contain pine essence. Working with pine wood and exposure to pine trees outdoors or indoors (Christmas trees) can also trigger asthma in a sensitive person.

Formaldehyde   Formaldehyde—a colorless, pungent, irritating gas—is a rare cause of occupational asthma. It is chiefly used as a disinfectant and preservative and in synthesizing other compounds, but it has a multitude of applications. It is used in the textile industry for hardening fibres; in the chemicals and plastics industries for the manufacture of melamine, formaldehyde resins, and celluloid; in the rubber industry for vulcanization processes; for the destruction of anthrax spores in wool, skins, and leather; as an embalming fluid; and as a bactericide and preservative of anatomical and pathological specimens.

Formaldehyde's irritation can extend beyond the workplace. People living in modern mobile homes that are extremely airtight, allowing for little inside air exchange, can be exposed to formaldehyde fumes, emitted from particle board, fibreboard, and plywood. Also on the home front, formaldehyde fumes can be emitted from the urea foam used in insulation materials.

Putting workplace and home-front exposure statistics in perspective, we find that 1.5 million workers and 11 million mobile-home dwellers are exposed to formaldehyde yearly. But, fortunately, only a very small minority of these people appears to develop asthma symptoms. Since its odor is so easily identified, formaldehyde is frequently blamed for causing asthma when the asthma has actually been caused by something else. Because of its irritating qualities, formaldehyde may aggravate asthma symptoms but it's usually not the source of the symptoms.

Dyes and Diazonium Salts Reactive dyes (azo and anthra quinone dyes), used in coloring cotton and synthetic fibres and used by hairdressers, and diazonium salts, widely used in photocopying, both have been incriminated for inducing occupational asthma. However, it is not positively known if they are responsible for significant amounts of occupational asthma. Azobisformamide, a relative to azo dyes, used as a foaming agent in the plastics industry, has also been implicated as a causative agent in occupational asthma. If these dyes and salts do induce asthma, it is probably through an allergic reaction.

Ethylenediamine and Paraphenylenediamine Ethylenediamine, used as an accelerator in the rubber industry and a solvent in the lacquer industry, and paraphenylenediamine, used in the fur industry, have both been incriminated as sources of occupational asthma. These substances probably induce asthma through an allergic reaction.

Others Some other chemical agents known to cause occupational asthma are:

- persulfates, used in bleaching agents by hairdressers;
- monethanolamine, used in nail spray and cold-wave permanent solutions;
- ammonium thioglycolate, sometimes found in wave-set lotions;
- hexamethylenetetramine, used as a paint thinner and in the manufacture of artificial resins;
- freon, used as a coolant in air-conditioning systems (causes asthma when heated);
- chloramine-t, used as a disinfectant in industry;
- tetrazene, used in the production of detonator caps;
- aminoethylethanolamine, a major ingredient in aluminum soldering flux; and
- carmine, a natural dye extracted from the insect *Coccus cactus*, used in the manufacture of cosmetics and biological dyes.

METAL SALTS

Occupational asthma is common among workers dealing with platinum salts, which are used in the manufacture of catalysts, in electroplating, in photography, in the production of fluorescent screens, and in jewelry and platinum refining. Asthma symptoms occur when the individual has contact with the dust of the salts of platinum (platinum combined with another element) and not with the dust of the elemental metal itself.

Platinum salts are possibly the most potent allergens to man. Evidence of their high sensitizing capacity is reflected in these statistics: An atopic person (one who easily develops allergy) develops sensitivity to platinum salts 100 percent of the time within 5 months of exposure, and at around 5 months after initial exposure sensitivity starts to occur even in nonatopic individuals. Fortunately, exposure to this allergen is very limited, and occurs almost exclusively in platinum-refinery workers and in chemists who use the salts. However, these workers can carry debris from the salts home on their clothing, thereby sensitizing the people in their living environment.

The following inorganic chemicals are occupational asthma culprits of a lesser degree: nickel, widely used in several industries; vanadium, used in the production of high-speed tools and photographic materials; chromium, found in stainless-steel welding fumes; and inhaled fumes from acids, alkalies, and gaseous halogens, such as bromine, chlorine, and fluorine.

DRUGS AND ENZYMES

Drugs Occupational asthma has occurred in workers involved in manufacturing or dispensing drugs, just as it has occurred in people who ingest the drugs. For workers—especially those who work in manufacturing—it's the inhalation of the powder or dust from the drugs and their derivatives that causes the asthma. Most reactions are allergic.

The following are some of the drugs suspected of causing asthma:

- penicillin-class drugs and a related class of drugs known as cephalosporins, which are common and widely used antibiotics;
- piperazine, used to treat worm infestations in animals and humans;
- cimetadine, an antihistamine, which works as an antacid in treating ulcers;
- psyllium, used as a bulk laxative;
- spiramycin, used as an antibiotic additive to poultry feed;
- aprolium hydrochloride, used as a poultry food additive and for preventing fungus infections;
- phenylglycine acid chloride, used in the manufacture of ampicillin, a common antibiotic;
- methyl dopa, a common antihypertensive drug; and
- tetracycline, a common antibiotic.

Enzymes Enzymes are complex proteins produced by living tissues, which catalyze or accelerate specific biochemical reactions. A variety of enzymes are capable of causing asthma upon inhalation. Atopic individuals (those more susceptible to allergy) are more readily affected than nonatopics. The following enzymes may be involved in causing asthma at the workplace:

- alcalase and maxatose, proteolytic enzymes (enzymes that break down proteins) derived from *Bacillus subtilis*, which have been widely used in the detergent washing-powder industry over the past several years. (These enzymes caused significant problems in the early-to-mid-1970s by plaguing exposed workers in the United States with asthma symptoms. As a result, the detergents were removed for a few years. However, they were recently reinstated in the form of a capsule, which has appreciably lessened exposure to the enzyme powder, resulting in less asthma. Along with the detergent industry, exposure to these enzymes may occur in the brewing, baking, silk, and leather industries.);

- pancreatic enzymes, which are used to improve digestion in people with pancreatic enzyme deficiency (asthma has also been reported in pharmacists dispensing pancreatic enzymes);

- pepsin, used as a digestive aid in medicine;

- papain, used mainly as a meat tenderizer, but also used to debride infected wounds and to clarify beer;

- bromelain, used as a meat tenderizer and in chill-proofing beer;

- trypsin, used in plastic polymer production, in debridement of wounds, and in medical treatment of thrombi (blood clots);

- flaviastase, used in various pharmaceuticals; and

- alpha-amylase, used in flour milling and the baking industry.

INSECTS, ANIMALS, AND FUNGI

Occupations that bring workers in contact with insect materials can prompt asthma, and the situation worsens when the contact takes place in poorly ventilated areas. Laboratory workers, fish-bait breeders, fishermen, mill workers, farm workers, bakers, and entomologists are people in these types of occupations. Asthma reactions resulting from inhalation of insect particles are usually allergic.

The list of insects reported to cause symptoms includes locusts, beetles, cockroaches, crickets, bee moths, flies, maggots, grain weevils, grain storage mites, moths, butterflies, and silk worms.

Exposure to animal materials is a common cause of asthma for veterinarians, stable hands, research workers, zoo keepers, kennel workers, and livestock and farm workers. The main allergen usually comes from the animal's skin dander, saliva, and blood particles—not from the animal's hair. Many kinds of animals are known to cause asthma in occupational settings, including horses, cattle, sheep, goats, hogs, rats, mice, guinea pigs, poultry, and domestic animals such as cats and dogs.

Sea squirt fluid (fluid from lower sea-life creatures attached to oysters), prawns, oysters, and pearl shell dust can cause allergic-triggered asthma for certain people, such as oyster gatherers and shuckers, prawn processors, and pearl shell openers.

Fungi and mould spores, common allergic triggers for asthma in the general population, can also result in occupational asthma. In bakers, asthma can result from inhalation of alternaria and aspergillus mould spores. Farm workers who come under heavy exposure to field mould spores are possible targets for asthma, as are cheese workers exposed to penicillium mould and chiropodists exposed to the fungi causing athlete's foot.

WOOD DUST

For years wood dusts were believed to act as nonspecific respiratory irritants, but it is now recognized that many woods are known to cause asthma, possibly through allergic reactions. The most reactive wood is Western red cedar, which is being used in increasing quantities in indoor and outdoor construction work. The agent responsible for asthma symptoms in Western red cedar is *plicatic acid.*

About 5 percent of the workers exposed to Western red cedar dust will develop asthma. The period of exposure to Western red cedar dust before symptoms occur is approximately 4 to 5 years. Asthma reactions may persist for days or weeks after cessation of exposure. Western red cedar dust may also produce a prolonged hyperreactive state of the airways, in which asthma symptoms persist for 3 to 4 years or even permanently. Nonsmoking workers appear to be more susceptible than smoking workers to developing Western red cedar asthma; the reason for this is not known. However, smoking workers with evidence of chronic bronchitis prior to the development of asthma from red cedar develop more permanent asthma symptoms.

Other woods that may contribute towards asthma at the workplace are oak, mahogany, mulberry, mansonia, cedar of Lebanon, California redwood, cocobolo, kajaat, African zebrawood, African maple, Quillaja bark (soap bark), Central American walnut, lauan, and iroko.

People associated with exposure to wood dusts are woodcarvers, wood finishers, woodworkers, carpenters, sawmillers, joiners, shingle millers, paper-mill workers, supply clerks, and numerous other workers who are directly or indirectly exposed.

GRAIN, PLANT DUSTS, AND VEGETABLE GUMS

Grain and its products contain many potent allergens. Not only is the grain protein itself allergenic, but contaminating substances found in the grain can be highly allergenic. These substances include wheat hairs, parasitic fungi (aspergillis, cladosporium, and aureobasidium), insects such as the grain weevil (Sitophilus granarius), and storage mites (Tyrophagus longior and Acarus farris)—all of which have been proven responsible for provoking asthma in exposed workers. All of these substances can make grain and grain dust highly allergenic. If someone is sensitive to one grain, he is usually sensitive to many types of grain. For instance, there is high cross-sensitivity between wheat and rye and their hybrid, triticale. The most common grains to which sensitization occurs are wheat, rye, barley, oats, and buckwheat. Atopic individuals (those more susceptible to allergy) are more likely to become sensitive than nonatopics.

Most people experiencing occupational asthma from grain-dust inhalation can ingest these grains without difficulty (except for buckwheat). This is probably because the allergenic portions of the grain are denatured during baking or they are destroyed by enzymatic digestion in the intestinal tract.

People likely to develop grain-dust-induced asthma from the workplace include millers, dockers, cooks and bakers, workers who transport grain products, farmers, and grain-elevator workers. In workers exposed to grain, the high prevalence of respiratory symptoms fluctuates with the intensity of their exposure to grain dust. For instance, dust levels in grain elevators can be extremely high—even up to several hundred milligrams per cubic metre of air. Fungal spores and storage mites that burrow into the stored grain are additional sensitizers. Studies show that work-related asthma symptoms occur in approximately 30 percent of all grain handlers and approximately 10 percent of all bakers (this is commonly known as "baker's asthma"). Some studies claim that not only asthma but chronic bronchitis may be related to prolonged grain-dust exposure, with cigarette smoking making these conditions worse.

Asthma from grain-dust inhalation is usually caused by an allergic reaction. Although asthma from grain dust is more common in atopic workers, it is not uncommon in nonatopic workers because the grain dust may cause a hyperreactive airway state that can lead to asthma upon exposure to other nonallergenic triggers.

Asthma related to occupational dust exposure is not limited to grain.

For many years exposure to castor beans has also been known to cause occupational asthma. Asthma can develop in workers involved in the production of castor-bean oil, in people who live near castor-bean mills, and in those using dried-bean residue as fertilizer.

Symptoms can also arise in workers in the coffee-bean industry, where people are exposed to the dust and chaff of green coffee beans. Some workers in the coffee-bean industry are exposed to castor-bean dust as well since both industries use the same sacks for transportation. Asthma from both castor beans and coffee beans is caused by an allergic reaction.

Other types of plant-dust-related asthma at the workplace include garlic-dust asthma, in those working in spice-processing plants; cinnamon-dust asthma, in those involved in harvesting and processing cinnamon bark; tea-fluff asthma, in workers exposed to the very fine tea dust that is discharged into the atmosphere during manufacturing and blending of tea; tobacco-dust asthma, in workers exposed to the green tobacco leaf; and hops asthma, in workers involved in the production of beer.

Similarly, occupational asthma due to exposure to dusts of vegetable gums, such as acacia, karaya, and tragacanth, has been reported in the color-printing trade. Since these gums are not used much in this trade anymore, the problem has diminished. Exposure to dusts of vegetable gums occasionally still causes problems for workers in the drug-manufacturing, candy-manufacturing, and food-processing industries.

BYSSINOSIS

Another type of occupational asthma due to plant-dust exposure is byssinosis. This asthma—caused by exposure to cotton, flax, or hemp dust—has been found in all countries of the world where these materials are spun and processed. Because it is associated with the onset of chest tightness in workers on Monday morning, it's commonly referred to as "Monday morning fever." It matters not in what geographic location the disease is found—the symptoms are always the same.

Symptoms typically include chest tightness and shortness of breath, which develop upon returning to work each Monday. The greatest risk of exposure and ensuing symptoms is associated with the manufacture of cotton yarn, and specifically with the cleaning process, known as carding. Carding involves the final removal of fibre impurities and the subsequent aligning of the fibres. Regardless of the differing processes and machines used, carding is always part of the process. After carding comes spinning, weaving, and finishing, all of which are relatively dust-free, thereby producing fewer symptoms.

It usually takes about 10 years of exposure before byssinosis begins to develop. When it does develop, its symptom patterns can be categorized into three different grades, based on severity:

1. chest tightness and/or shortness of breath on only the first day of the work week (these symptoms are reversible when exposure ceases),

2. chest tightness and/or shortness of breath on the first few days of the work week (these symptoms are reversible when exposure ceases), and

3. chest tightness and/or shortness of breath on every day of the work week (these prolonged symptoms tend to become irreversible and occur almost exclusively in smokers).

The prevalence of byssinosis among cotton-mill workers ranges anywhere from 17 to 38 percent. The prevalence increases when workers smoke, and smoking may be the sole cause for the irreversible component associated with the grade-three symptom patterns noted earlier.

How byssinosis develops is unclear. Allergy plays no role. Studies have revealed the major offending agent to be in the bract, the leaflike structure enfolding the cotton boll.

Improved ventilation, proper maintenance of equipment, and improved dust-reducing processing techniques have been helpful in decreasing the development of byssinosis. But it is still advisable that people who smoke not work in industries related to byssinosis because they may develop an irreversible respiratory component that will not yield to treatment.

How Is Asthma at the Workplace Diagnosed?

If you suspect asthma related to your workplace, it's best to take the problem to an allergist.

The allergist will first take a medical history, with emphasis on the nature and type of exposure to potential causative agents for workplace-induced asthma. He will place special emphasis on the onset, severity, and duration of your asthma symptoms in relation to exposure at your workplace.

Next, he will administer a bronchodilator pulmonary function test or a methacholine pulmonary function test to confirm a diagnosis of asthma.

After the presence of asthma is confirmed, determining suspected occupational allergic triggers follows. This is done by skin testing or RAST testing, if the suspected material is available for testing. However, the single, most convincing diagnostic test for asthma at the workplace is the *bronchial provocation challenge test.* Bronchial provocation testing with different agents found in the work environment can aid in identifying the causative agent. Unfortunately, these provocation tests are time-consuming and technical and, at least in the United States, are only available at a few medical centers. Therefore, a simpler procedure is often used involving pulmonary function measurements before, during, and after work to document the association between asthma and the workplace. This can be done with a portable spirometer or peak flowmeter. (For more information on asthma testing methods, see Chapter 5.)

If an occupational cause for your asthma is suspected, a trial period away from your workplace or a temporary change to another job area at your workplace may be necessary. Then, if your symptoms go away, a trial period back at your workplace is in order to see if your symptoms will return. If so, it would suggest an occupational cause for your asthma.

What Other Lung Conditions Besides Asthma Can Be Caused by the Workplace?

Not all occupational lung conditions caused by the workplace are asthma; harmful agents in the workplace can injure lungs in various ways, resulting in other respiratory diseases. Some nonasthmatic lung conditions related to the workplace are:

- coal worker's pneumoconiosis (black lung disease), caused from inhaling coal dust;
- silicosis, caused from inhaling crystalline silica;
- asbestosis, caused from inhaling asbestos fibres;
- berylliosis, caused by inhaling beryllium; and
- hypersensitive pneumonitis, an immune reaction in the lungs, resulting from inhaling certain kinds of small mould spores or other proteins, which includes a myriad of conditions—such as farmer's lung, pigeon breeder's disease, cheese worker's lung, mushroom worker's lung, bagasosis (in sugar-cane workers), suberosis (in cork workers), and sequoiosis (in woodworkers).

We mention these conditions to increase your awareness of common occupational lung diseases that aren't due to airway hyperreactivity as asthma is. Rather, they are due to inflammation and scarring of the air sacs and the tissue between the air sacs and the lung capillaries, as a result of inhalation of various dust fumes and particles found in some workplace environments.

What Can Be Done To Treat Occupational Asthma?

Of course, removing the asthmatic from the workplace would be a sure way to eliminate problems, but this is not always a realistic or even workable solution. Medical treatment then becomes the best measure to keep the asthmatic as symptom-free as possible. With use of the proper medications, satisfactory control is often possible for many asthmatics (this is discussed in detail in Chapter 8). However, there are individuals who are severely reactive to occupational agents causing asthma. When medical treatment has been tried and has failed for these people, the only realistic solution would be removal from the workplace.

What Can Be Done To Prevent Occupational Asthma?

Prevention rather than treatment is the ultimate goal in the management of occupational asthma. To achieve results, prevention and control must include efforts to educate workers and employers in high-risk industries. They must learn to recognize potential occupational asthma hazards in their work environments. Once recognition is achieved, industries can work towards reducing contact with potentially harmful agents by monitoring employees yearly for asthma symptoms, improving ventilation and cleanliness standards to ensure dust and fume control, and improving safety measures in disposing of harmful agents. These are realistic, workable preventive measures that can benefit the employer and the employee. Also, in a few high-risk industries, it may be in the employer's and employees' best interest not to hire workers with atopy (allergy) or underlying asthma, or those who smoke.

Finally, people in government agencies, the medical field, and industries must continue to work together in reducing and/or eliminating occupational asthma in the workplace. Only then can we have safe, healthy workers who can be productive and remain asthma-free.

15
Stress, Hyperventilation, and Asthma

Let's begin by dispelling a long-standing myth: Asthma is *not* a psychological or emotional disease. Fortunately, both doctors and patients have finally come to realize the danger in that old myth. Believing that asthma is a disease caused by a psychological problem closes the door on discovering its real cause and often interferes with treatment. However, asthma does have a real, not imagined, association with our emotions. What's the connection? Human feelings of fear, depression, guilt, panic, pleasurable excitement, and joy, to name a few. Yes, all of these emotions can provoke asthma because they all can cause stress.

Let's examine the relationship between stress and asthma more closely by taking a look at one day in the life of an asthmatic named Bonnie, a competent, conscientious business administrator as well as an attentive and loving wife and mother. Bonnie's day started off with a boom. She overslept and had to get herself and her family going in record time so that the kids would get to school and she would get to an important staff meeting on time. To make matters worse, her husband was out of town, so he couldn't share in getting things moving. One of the kids couldn't find his field-trip permission slip he'd just remembered was due that morning and he started crying. Bonnie searched, but to no avail, so she had to write an impromptu note, while she tried to comfort her upset son. Readying herself and her kids for the day took a lot of extra energy, causing Bonnie to feel a bit zapped as she raced through rush-hour traffic to the office. In her haste, she left some important corporate papers at home that she needed for her meeting. She quickly grabbed her preliminary notes to use in their place. Although she made it through her meeting adequately, she felt disorganized and frazzled. She began feeling the familiar chest tightness she recognized as a symptom of asthma, but she wasn't coughing or wheezing and she didn't have a cold, so she assumed she was just feeling the pressures of the hectic morning.

The afternoon seemed to follow suit from her morning: Her clients met her with numerous demands; a couple of promising business possibilities went sour; her husband phoned to say he would be detained another day; and the secretary at school called in midafternoon, saying she must come and get her daughter, who had cut her knee on the playground at recess and appeared to need stitches. She made quick arrangements with her secretary to handle things for the rest of the afternoon at the office, and left to pick up her daughter and take her to the hospital emergency ward. While waiting at the hospital and trying to comfort her daughter, she remembered she needed to call her baby-sitter to tell her not to expect her daughter after school. The woman would be thinking that the child had been kidnapped!

By the time she finally got both kids home, fed, bathed, and in bed, she felt sick. Her chest symptoms were increasing and she felt she could not get enough air. She panicked and began to feel as though she were suffocating. She had never experienced such severe asthma. She phoned her physician, who, after listening to Bonnie, assured her that her symptoms were probably triggered by hyperventilation. He told her that hyperventilation means over-breathing, and that it's a common response to stress made by many asthmatics. He prescribed her usual medication (which she had on hand, thank goodness!), and told her to come see him tomorrow to talk about ways to cope with asthma triggered by hyperventilation and stress.

Bonnie could have effectively coped with and modified her responses to the common triggers that had provoked her asthma, but she didn't realize it. Why? Probably because she never really associated asthma with stress or hyperventilation.

What Is Stress?

We seem to hear a lot about stress nowadays. It pops up as a favorite topic in many popular magazines, on various health-related talk shows, and in casual conversation. People are concerned about stress, and well they should be, especially since stress appears to be the universal angst of our time! What is stress? Very simply, stress is your body's automatic response to any demand made upon it. The events or circumstances that create stress are called *stressors* (remember Bonnie and all her stressors?).

Stress is an unavoidable fact of life, and it isn't all bad. Some stress is good because it gets you "in gear" to face life's challenges (as when you are delivering a speech) or gives you that spurt of energy to finish an important project. But too much stress is bad; it frazzles your nerves and wreaks havoc with your emotions. What's more, too much stress can make you miserable and ill.

Actually, stress is a legacy from our prehistoric ancestors. In prehistoric times, stress was the caveman's response to the warning snap of a twig outside the cave. This response, known as "fight or flight," prepared our early ancestors to fight or flee from daily life-threatening situations. The response was involuntary. Today we respond to stress with the same basic fight or flight response, though we're seldom faced with dangers similar to our ancestors'. Yet our bodies respond to stress involuntarily as though we are fighting for our lives or are about to flee when we react to modern daily stressors, such as financial problems, deadlines, arguments, and traffic jams. Responding to these acute stressors usually results in short-term, easily identified stress. However, complex family and/or personal problems or health problems that persist over a long period of time can result in chronic stress, which is often difficult to identify.

We all experience stress—good and bad—in varying degrees, but asthmatics are especially vulnerable to stress. Read on to find out why.

What Happens Inside When We Experience Stress?

Bonnie's day illustrates the link between the emotional responses of worry, fear, and anxiety and the physical reactions we associate with stress.

Consider this scene: You are leaving your job late one evening. You are walking alone to your car in a large, deserted parking lot. Everything is quiet. Suddenly you hear footsteps behind you and you are several rows away from your car. This is what takes place in your body: Your brain sends signals to your adrenal gland, which then secretes adrenaline. This makes your heart beat faster; you feel a rush of energy. Your blood flow increases and is directed from your skin and stomach to your muscles, preparing them for fight or flight. Sugars are released into the blood stream for quick energy. Your breathing rate increases, pupils dilate, and muscles tense and tighten.

But as an asthmatic, your increased breathing rate causes you to overbreathe, or hyperventilate (more about this later), and your hyperreactive airways are prime targets for the tension and constriction associated with stress.

What Causes Stress?

Any demands or changes in our work life, family life, or day-to-day living—be they subtle or drastic—can bring about stress. It all depends on how you perceive the situation and respond to it. Some people thrive on confrontation, whereas confrontation makes others physically ill. A young mother facing new demands and responsibilities can feel the effects of stress just as readily and to as great an extent as a corporate president facing multimillion-dollar decisions. Whatever the stressor, if it creates stress for you it is real and should be dealt with before it deals with you.

What Are Common Signs and Symptoms of Stress?

Stress affects us emotionally and physically. Here are some common signs and symptoms of stress:

- cold hands and feet
- frequent jaw clenching
- muscle tension
- light-headedness
- muscle aches and pains
- fatigue
- palpitations
- general loss of interest in life
- recurrent diarrhea and/or constipation
- sensation of shortness of breath with or without a feeling of a lump in your throat

- dry mouth
- nervousness
- listlessness
- frequent headaches
- heartburn
- feeling of depression
- frequent crying
- changes in: sleeping patterns, eating habits, and sexual habits

Recognize any of these? If you do, you probably are feeling the effects of stress. If you are an asthmatic, take heed. Stress could be triggering your asthma, or another condition that causes shortness of breath known as hyperventilation.

What Is Hyperventilation and How Is It Related to Asthma and to Stress?

Hyperventilation, very simply, means over-breathing in relation to your body's metabolic needs. It occurs when you increase your rate and volume of breathing beyond the metabolic requirement.

Basically, hyperventilation is a habit of poor breathing, which people fail to recognize in themselves. It is similar to someone having poor posture for so long he doesn't recognize it. As an asthmatic, you must control your breathing habits to guard against hyperventilation, which, in itself, can trigger an asthma attack.

For a closer look at hyperventilation and asthma, let's consider Jim, a 35-year-old asthmatic, who was eagerly and conscientiously starting a new restaurant business. He had spent many hours working on organizing, planning, ordering, hiring, and all the unavoidable legal aspects of his business. While excited and challenged by the new venture, he was also anxious and tense about the risk. He had a nagging fear that maybe he couldn't make a go of it. In response to his anxiety, fear, and tension, he hyperventilated. He felt constantly short of breath and tight-chested. On top of that, lately he'd been feeling light-headed and his fingers kept tingling. Then his asthma flared and a vicious cycle of stress, hyperventilation, and asthma ensued.

When Jim hyperventilated, he was breathing by mainly using his upper-chest and neck muscles. He was taking shallow and quick breaths. He was so tense even his breathing was tense. His symptoms of shortness of breath and light-headedness were typical of hyperventilation. These and other hyperventilation symptoms he could have experienced are highlighted in the list that follows. All of these symptoms occur because the rapid breathing results in carbon dioxide "blowing off," which causes a decrease in the circulation of blood to the brain and an increase in the release of oxygen to the body tissues.

Common Signs and Symptoms of Hyperventilation

• Shortness of breath	• Frequent sighing
• Chest tightness and/or pain	• Tremors
• Light-headedness	• Dry mouth
• Numbness around mouth	• Palpitations
• Tingling of fingers and toes	• Fatigue

How Can I Tell If I'm Hyperventilating?

You can tell if you have a problem with hyperventilation by consciously making yourself hyperventilate to see if you can reproduce some of the symptoms, but you really don't need to subject yourself to this. Instead, why not try noticing your general breathing patterns, paying special attention to your stomach, chest, and neck areas. Your stomach should move out with inspiration and in with expiration if you are breathing correctly (refer to the section on "Relaxed Breathing" on page 183), and your chest and neck should move only slightly. Take time now to notice your breathing.

Other than becoming aware of your breathing patterns, the best way to detect if you have a problem with hyperventilation is to go to your doctor and discuss it with him.

How Are Stress, Hyperventilation, and Asthma Related?

Asthmatics—even when they are not under stress and do not have any asthma symptoms—are prone to hyperventilation. The hyperventilation is often subtle with frequent sighing respirations and upper-chest breathing.

Hyperventilation occurs in asthmatics because of a persistence of small airway narrowing in their lungs, even when they are not experiencing asthma. The small airway narrowing causes stimulation of nerve receptors in the bronchial muscles, which in turn stimulate the respiratory center in the brain to cause rapid and deeper breathing.

Stress, from *any* source, can stimulate the sympathetic nervous system to increase a person's rate of breathing. This naturally will worsen any underlying hyperventilation tendency in an asthmatic. Hyperventilating decreases carbon dioxide in the blood, which in turn increases bronchospasms and worsens asthma. Asthma then becomes a stressor and causes the stress response.

The following illustration depicts the interrelationship among stress, hyperventilation, and asthma. Each of these conditions can worsen the others.

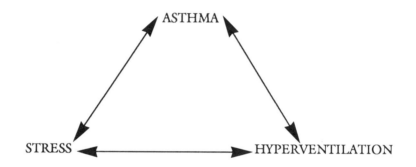

The best way to break this vicious cycle is through control and management of hyperventilation and stress. If you can get an edge on those two ends of the triangle, you can begin to take an active part in controlling your own asthma.

How Can the Hyperventilation, Stress, and Asthma Cycle Be Controlled?

You have the first step towards control at your fingertips: You now have an understanding of stress and hyperventilation, and of their relationship to asthma. But where do you go from here? First of all, see your doctor. Show him this chapter and discuss the relationship between stress, hyperventilation, and asthma, as it applies to you and your life. He may want to prescribe various asthma medications to control your asthma. Also, he may want to prescribe a mild tranquillizer for you as an anti-anxiety agent to help decrease your respiratory drive.

In addition to possible medications, there are other ways that you can alter your breathing response and reduce anxiety, tension, stress, and hyperventilation. These measures are easy to follow, cost nothing, and can be done in the privacy of your own home, or if suitable on your job. No method is necessarily better than another; which one will work for you is a matter of personal preference and positive results.

Try them. They only require your concentration, effort, desire to change, and practice. You'd be surprised how easily these techniques can become a part of your everyday life. Doing them for very short periods of time at the first signs of stress may be all you will need to thwart a full-blown alarm response. Anyway, you have nothing to lose besides some unwanted stress-response patterns.

RELAXED BREATHING

Relaxing your breathing is a good way to set the stage for totally relaxing your mind and body, and it is a good relaxation technique in its own right. There are many breathing-relaxation techniques available today and they all strive for the same goal: to help you relax.

There is a right and wrong way to breathe. The wrong way is known as *chest-stress breathing*, where you use upper-chest muscles mostly and take rapid, shallow breaths. This type of breathing stimulates the sympathetic nervous system, producing a widespread stress response, which often results in hyperventilation, asthma, and more stress.

The right way to breathe is known as *belly breathing*, whereby you breathe with your diaphragm (the main muscle for breathing, just under your rib cage), as you draw air clear down past your chest into your stomach. Examine your breathing pattern. Are you a chest-breather or a belly-breather?

If you practise belly breathing, eventually you'll learn to respond to emotional stress and hyperventilation by breathing this way rather than going into a panic reaction. Practise this technique for 5 to 10 minutes several times a day:

1.   Sit up straight or lie down. Place one hand on your chest and the other on your stomach (this will help you "feel" how to inhale into your stomach instead of your chest).

2.   Inhale slowly and deeply through your nose, aiming for the bottom of your stomach. Feel your stomach swell out as you slowly pull air in (the hand on your stomach should rise; the hand on your chest should hardly rise).

3.   Then exhale slowly through your mouth. You should feel your stomach pull in and flatten.

4.   Repeat the process slowly and evenly.

You may want to add *visualization* to your relaxed breathing. Close your eyes. Picture a quiet, calm place. For instance, think of the ocean moving in and out on a warm shoreline. See the place in your mind. Breathe in with the waves and breathe out with the waves. Picture your tension flowing from your body, leaving you loose. Visualizing can soothe your mind, help release tension, and aid in breathing relaxation.

When you're under pressure or starting to hyperventilate, rely on the calming effects of relaxed breathing. Also, remember to make a conscious effort to belly-breathe whenever you can, until it becomes your normal breathing pattern. Practise daily for the best results.

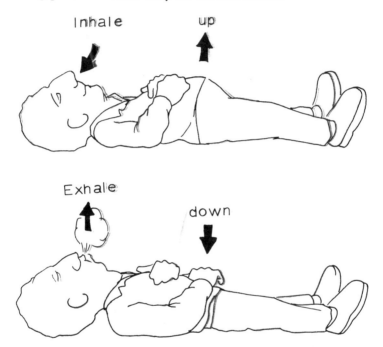

This drawing shows the proper technique to use for relaxed breathing (diaphragmatic breathing). Note how the abdomen rises with the inhale and flattens with the exhale while the chest barely moves.

PROGRESSIVE MUSCLE RELAXATION

You can use this technique to relax yourself and rid your muscles of stress: Sit or lie down in a quiet place. Begin by doing some relaxed breathing (even five or six relaxed inhales and exhales will set the stage). You will be tensing and then relaxing different muscle groups in your body, one at a time. (Tense for 5 to 7 seconds, relax for 10 seconds.) As you progress through the muscle groups, try *visualizing* the tension flowing from your muscles or say to yourself "I am letting tension go." It doesn't matter if you start with your head or your feet, but do each muscle group separately:

- feet and ankles
- calves
- thighs
- buttocks
- abdomen
- hands
- arms
- shoulders
- neck
- face
(tense all facial muscles, wrinkle forehead, clench jaws)

You should feel loose and relaxed when you're finished. Notice this feeling. This exercise is particularly good in helping you learn to notice the difference between the feeling of tension and the feeling of relaxation in your muscle groups. With practice, you should be able to quickly identify muscle tension, and then you can start relaxing to combat it.

BIOFEEDBACK

As we stated, knowing the difference between being tense and being relaxed is important in moderating your stress response. Biofeedback is a great way to learn the difference and to help make you aware of subtle stress signals in your body. Contrary to the popular notion, biofeedback doesn't alter your body's stress state; it is simply a method used to identify and measure your body's stress level.

During biofeedback you are hooked up to a machine that reads changes in your brain waves, muscle tension, or skin temperature (each of these is an indirect measurement of your stress state). These measurements are relayed to you by a beeping sound. The more beeps, the more stressed you are. When you relax, the beep slows down. Your job is to recognize the feeling of relaxation as you feel it and "hear" it measured on the biofeedback machine.

To be most effective, biofeedback is usually used in conjunction with other relaxation techniques to help you discover and cope with your stress responses.

You can buy inexpensive biofeedback tools to use at home to help you control your stress response. Proven studies have demonstrated positive results with the use of progressive muscle relaxation and biofeedback in controlling asthma—especially with asthmatics who experience the anxiety, panic, and fear reflective of both stress and hyperventilation.

MEDITATION

Another method used to combat the body's stress response is meditation. Meditation works well because, besides increasing a feeling of overall relaxation and well-being, it lowers respiration and heart rate, decreases blood pressure, and reduces body metabolism.

To meditate you need a quiet place and a comfortable environment. Use relaxed breathing (belly breathing) and relax your muscles. Each time you breathe out slowly, say a calming word to yourself, such as "one" or "peace." Concentrating on this word will help you block out all other thoughts. Continue for about 15 minutes.

As with any other relaxation technique, to have it work for you means you need to practise. Your meditation will get easier as you integrate it into your life.

GENERAL DE-STRESSORS TO EASE YOUR LIFE

Here are some general suggestions for making your life more stress-free and hopefully more asthma-free when stress is the culprit.

Exercise regularly This can be a great outlet for stress and a wonderful energizer. Try it.

Talk it over Talk out your problems with a friend or someone you trust who will listen to you. If you have no one in whom to confide, talk to a minister or counsellor. Sometimes just getting things "off your chest" can relieve stress.

Get enough rest and sleep Nerves tend to fray when you're tired. No matter how busy you are, never cut back on your sleep. The more rested you are, the better you can face your world.

Take time out Be good to yourself. Every day take some time just for yourself—to read, relax, or be alone with your thoughts. Also, get away for a vacation with your friends or loved ones. Nothing is as rejuvenating as a change of scenery and some fun.

Manage your time better When your responsibilities seem endless, stress really mounts. Plan your work and errands to avoid feeling overwhelmed. Don't forget to plan time for enjoyment. Try to get up 30 minutes earlier in the morning to enjoy breakfast and not rush.

Learn to say no It's okay to say no. Drop activities you don't enjoy, and don't accept more work than you can handle.

Express your feelings If you're angry, say so. Suppressing your feelings only bottles them up and creates monumental stress. If you need to cry, then do! Crying is a way of letting off steam and letting go of intense feelings.

Take time to realize the joy in your life The little joys of life are important stress reducers. If you take time out to experience some of the simple pleasures available to you, you may suffer less asthma. For instance, spend some time with your family. Go out to dinner. Enjoy a good relationship with your spouse, lover, and friends.

Visualize We mentioned this earlier in conjunction with other relaxation techniques, but it is actually a relaxer in its own right. All you need is your imagination and to let yourself daydream to bring yourself to a peaceful place from your past or even to a place where you've never been. Besides making you feel good, daydreaming can also prepare you for a stress-provoking situation. If you know a situation is going to occur that will provoke stress and trigger your asthma, visualize the event and rehearse what you can do to make it less stressful. Visualize yourself responding in a relaxed, calm manner. Positive visualization can be a powerful tool in helping you control the stress that can cause your asthma. See if it works for you.

Believe in yourself Realize that you alone can minimize your stress and hyperventilation, control your asthma, and make your life better. Others can only give you advice for a stress-free life. You must take the advice and integrate it into your life so that it works for you.

o   o   o

Take a close look at your asthma. Is it triggered by stress and hyperventilation? How often do you experience the emotions associated with stress and hyperventilation—anger, tension, fear, anxiety, panic, or excitability? Daily? If you experience any of these emotions frequently, and if you are an asthmatic, there is undoubtedly an association between your asthma symptoms and your stress response. Recognize your stress responses, talk to your doctor about medications, and listen to your body when it signals asthma. You don't have to live with the vicious stress-hyperventilation-asthma cycle; you can break free of it with awareness, understanding, and action. Let this chapter inspire you to start coping with and controlling your stress-related asthma triggers today.

Appendices

Appendix A
The Respiratory System and How It Works

Our respiratory system is responsible for our breathing and is concerned with the gaseous interchange between our body and its environment.

Basically, breathing is the process by which we inhale (breathe air in) and exhale (breathe air out). The specific terms that apply to breathing are *inspiration*, meaning to draw in, and *expiration*, meaning to release. This procedure of inhaling and exhaling as a single, complete act of breathing is called *respiration*. While resting, the average person breathes approximately 12 to 16 times per minute and takes in about a pint of air with each inhalation. We breathe without thinking about it while we are sleeping, playing, and working.

What Is the Basic Function of the Respiratory System?

The basic function of the respiratory system is to provide the oxygen necessary for the essential processes of body metabolism and to rid the body of carbon-dioxide waste. Since oxygen and carbon dioxide are gases, this process is called gas exchange.

Oxygen composes 21 percent of the air we breathe; the remaining 79 percent is composed of nitrogen and other gases in trace amounts. Air contains less than .03 percent carbon dioxide. Oxygen is necessary to sustain life, whereas carbon dioxide must be removed from the blood to maintain life. If breathing is less than adequate, not enough oxygen will be made available to our body tissues for them to perform properly; furthermore, carbon dioxide, the waste product of tissue function, will build to toxic levels.

The functioning of the entire respiratory system is coordinated and regulated by parts of our central nervous system. We breathe when the brain sends impulses to the chest muscles and diaphragm to take in air. The rate of breathing is regulated by the respiratory center in the brain.

What Are the Components of the Respiratory System?

THE NOSE, LARYNX, AND TRACHEA (THE UPPER-RESPIRATORY SYSTEM)

Air is drawn into the body through the nose, which filters, moistens, and warms it. Lining the nasal wall is a thin membrane with tiny hairlike projections, called cilia. This membrane is rich in glands that produce a sticky secretion, called mucus. Mucus provides several functions: It possesses an acidic nature, which makes it unfavorable for the growth of bacteria and viruses; it forms a sticky surface to entrap dust and various foreign particles that are potentially harmful to our airway passages; and it aids the cilia in sweeping the various foreign particles to the back of the throat, where they can be harmlessly swallowed.

Air passes from the nasal area to the pharynx, in the upper part of the throat, and then on to the larynx, commonly known as our voice box, which is the narrowest part of the upper-respiratory system. The larynx is lined with mucous membranes and is composed of cartilage and cords, which are moved by sensitive muscles. Besides speech, important functions of the larynx are controlling air flow into our airways and acting as a valve in closing the entrance to the trachea in protection against foreign particles entering our airways.

Continuing on its passage, air then moves to the trachea, the passage leading from the larynx to the lungs. The trachea is composed of horseshoe-shaped cartilage rings. This flexible tube begins just below the larynx at the middle of the neck and runs to the upper third of the chest, where it divides into the right and left bronchial tubes (windpipes). This division, known as the carina, separates the upper- and lower-respiratory system.

THE LUNGS AND BRONCHIAL TUBES (THE LOWER-RESPIRATORY SYSTEM)

The lungs are located in the chest cavity; nestled between the lungs lies the heart. The right lung is divided into three lobes, or sections, and weighs approximately 625 grams, or just less than $1\frac{1}{2}$ pounds. The smaller left lung weighs approximately 565 grams, or about $1\frac{1}{4}$ pounds. Each lobe is similar to a balloon filled with soft, spongelike lung tissue. Bronchial tubes (windpipes) branch off from the right and left main bronchial tubes and go to each lobe, where they subdivide and branch further.

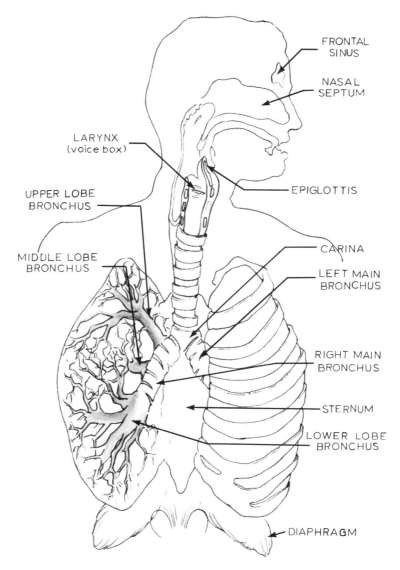

FRONTAL
SINUS

NASAL
SEPTUM

LARYNX
(voice box)

EPIGLOTTIS

UPPER LOBE
BRONCHUS

CARINA

LEFT MAIN
BRONCHUS

MIDDLE LOBE
BRONCHUS

RIGHT MAIN
BRONCHUS

STERNUM

LOWER LOBE
BRONCHUS

DIAPHRAGM

The respiratory system's important anatomical structures.

Our spongelike lung tissue consists of a system of branching windpipes, which are subdivided many times into tiny windpipes, called bronchioles. Lining the windpipes is a membrane with cilia, similar to that found in the nasal passage. Mucus produced in the windpipe walls catches and holds much of the dust, foreign particles, and other unwanted matter that has invaded the lungs. With a wavelike motion, the cilia carry the sticky mucus upwards and out to the throat, where it is either coughed up or swallowed.

Located at the end of the tiny bronchioles (the smallest of windpipes) are the alveoli; these are minute, grapelike clusters of air sacs. The alveoli are the destination of the air we breathe.

There are normally over 300,000,000 alveoli in both lungs. Alveoli walls are made of a thin membrane, through which the exchange between the oxygen of the air and the carbon dioxide of the blood takes place. This process is called the exchange of gases.

Each minute, while resting, we breathe approximately 6 litres, or about $1\frac{1}{3}$ gallons, of fresh air. About a third of it stays in our upper airways, while the remaining four litres (about one gallon) is distributed to the millions of tiny alveoli.

What Happens During the Exchange of Gases?

The main functions of the lungs are taking oxygen from the air that is inhaled and ridding the body of carbon dioxide that has been brought to the lungs by the blood stream. To accomplish the exchange of gases, air

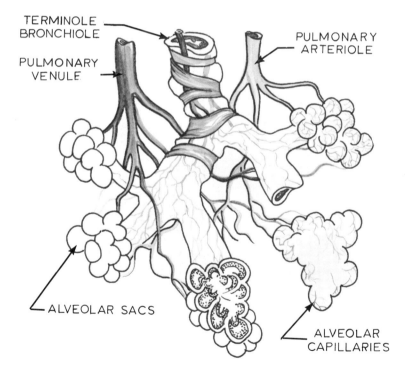

In this drawing, the respiratory system meets the circulatory system. Air passes through the terminole bronchioles to the alveolar sacs, where the exchange of oxygen and carbon dioxide takes place with the circulation.

EXCHANGE OF GASES

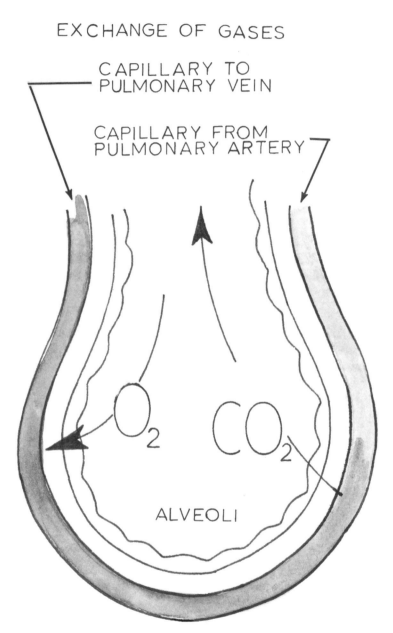

CAPILLARY TO
PULMONARY VEIN

CAPILLARY FROM
PULMONARY ARTERY

O_2

CO_2

ALVEOLI

This drawing of the exchange of gases depicts carbon dioxide coming from the pulmonary artery to the alveoli (air sacs) and oxygen going from the alveoli to the pulmonary vein.

is delivered to the alveoli. During the exchange, oxygen from the air spreads across the membranes into tiny blood capillaries embedded in the walls of the alveoli. Blood passes through the capillaries (brought to them by the pulmonary artery and taken away by the pulmonary vein). Each minute our heart pumps about 5 litres, or $1^1/_4$ gallons, of blood through the capillaries around the alveoli. While the blood is in the capillaries, it discharges carbon dioxide into the alveoli and takes up oxygen from the air in the alveoli. The cycle continues throughout the process of breathing.

How Do We Breathe?

Breathing depends upon the alteration of the volume of the chest cavity. Inspiration occurs when air is breathed into the body. This is accomplished when the chest expands and develops a negative air pressure within the chest cavity. Since the air pressure in the lungs is less than the atmospheric air pressure, air is literally forced into the lungs by the higher atmospheric air pressure. Expiration occurs when the chest contracts and thereby forces air out of the lungs into the atmosphere.

Breathing involves the muscles of the chest wall and the diaphragm. The diaphragm lies under the lungs and separates the chest cavity from the abdominal cavity. When relaxed the diaphragm is shaped like a dome. As nerve impulses signal our bodies to inhale, the diaphragm contracts and moves downwards to a flattened position, thus increasing the size of the chest cavity and enabling air to enter the lungs. While the diaphragm is contracting downwards, the muscles of the chest wall pull the chest cavity outward to further enlarge it for greater capacity during inhalation. During exhalation the reverse action occurs. The diaphragm moves upwards and pushes air out of the lungs by means of its muscle action. As the diaphragm moves upwards, the chest muscles move the chest cavity inward to help the diaphragm push air out.

Appendix B
Pollens Causing Allergy, and Where They're Found in the United States and Canada

NORTH ATLANTIC UNITED STATES

Connecticut	New Hampshire	Pennsylvania
Maine	New Jersey	Rhode Island
Massachusetts	New York	Vermont

Trees (Pollinating Season—Late Winter through Spring)

ash	cottonwood/poplar	oak
birch	elm	pine
box elder/maple	hickory	sycamore

Grasses (Pollinating Season—Spring through Early Summer)

bluegrass/June grass	orchard	Timothy
fescue	redtop	

Weeds (Pollinating Season—Summer through Early Fall)

cocklebur	lamb's quarters	ragweed—giant and
dock/sorrel	plantain	short

MID-ATLANTIC UNITED STATES

Delaware	Maryland	Virginia
District of Columbia	North Carolina	

Trees (Pollinating Season—Late Winter through Spring)

ash	cottonwood/poplar	mulberry
birch	elm	oak
box elder/maple	hackberry	walnut
cedar/juniper	hickory/pecan	

Grasses (Pollinating Season—Spring through Early Summer)

Bermuda grass	orchard grass	Timothy
bluegrass/June grass	redtop	vernal grass
Johnson grass	ryegrass	

Weeds (Pollinating Season—Summer through Early Fall)

cocklebur	Mexican firebush	ragweed—giant and
dock/sorrel	pigweed	short
lamb's quarters	plantain	

SOUTH ATLANTIC UNITED STATES

Florida, northern (above Orlando)	Georgia	South Carolina

Trees (Pollinating Season—Late Winter through Spring)

ash	cottonwood/poplar	mesquite
birch	elm	mulberry
box elder/maple	hackberry	oak
cedar/juniper	hickory/pecan	walnut

Grasses (Pollinating Season—Spring through Early Summer)

Bermuda grass	Johnson grass	ryegrass
bluegrass/June grass	orchard grass	Timothy
fescue	redtop	vernal grass

Weeds (Pollinating Season—Summer through Early Fall)

cocklebur	lamb's quarters	ragweed—giant and
dock/sorrel	plantain	short
		sagebrush

SUBTROPIC FLORIDA

Florida, southern (below Orlando)

Trees (Pollinating Season—Winter through Spring)

Australian pine (beefwood)	cedar/juniper	pecan
	cottonwood/poplar	privet
bayberry (wax myrtle)	elm	sycamore
box elder	melaleuca	
Brazilian peppertree (Florida holly)	oak	
	palm	

Grasses (Pollinating Season—Spring through Early Summer)

Bahia grass	canary grass	salt grass
Bermuda grass	Johnson grass	
bluegrass/June grass	redtop	

Weeds (Pollinating Season—Summer through Early Fall)

dock/sorrel	pigweed	sagebrush

lamb's quarters	plantain
marsh elder/	ragweed—giant and short
poverty weed	

THE GREATER OHIO VALLEY

| Indiana | Ohio | West Virginia |
| Kentucky | Tennessee | |

Trees (Pollinating Season—Late Winter through Spring

ash	cottonwood/poplar	oak
birch	elm	sycamore
box elder/maple	hickory	walnut

Grasses (Pollinating Season—Spring through Early Summer)

Bermuda grass	Johnson grass	ryegrass
bluegrass/June grass	orchard grass	Timothy
fescue	redtop	

Weeds (Pollinating Season—Summer through Early Fall)

cocklebur	plantain	sagebrush
dock/sorrel	ragweed—giant and	water hemp
lamb's quarters	short	
pigweed		

SOUTH CENTRAL UNITED STATES

| Alabama | Louisiana | Mississippi |
| Arkansas | | |

Trees (Pollinating Season—Late Winter through Spring)

ash	elm	sycamore
box elder/maple	hackberry	walnut
cedar/juniper	hickory/pecan	
cottonwood/poplar	oak	

Grasses (Pollinating Season—Spring through Early Summer)

Bermuda grass	orchard grass	Timothy
bluegrass/June grass	redtop	
Johnson grass	ryegrass	

Weeds (Pollinating Season—Summer through Early Fall)

careless weed/	lamb's quarters	ragweed—giant and
pigweed	marsh elder/	short
cocklebur	poverty weed	sagebrush
dock/sorrel	plantain	

THE NORTHERN MIDWEST

| Michigan | Minnesota | Wisconsin |

Trees (Pollinating Season—Late Winter through Spring)

alder	cottonwood/poplar	sycamore
ash	elm	walnut
birch	hickory	
box elder/maple	oak	

Grasses (Pollinating Season—Spring through Early Summer)

bluegrass/June grass	fescue	ryegrass
brome	orchard grass	Timothy
canary grass	redtop	

Weeds (Pollinating Season—Summer through Early Fall)

cocklebur	marsh elder/poverty	ragweed—giant
dock/sorrel	weed	and short
lamb's quarters	pigweed	Russian thistle
	plantain	water hemp

THE CENTRAL MIDWEST

Illinois	Iowa	Missouri

Trees (Pollinating Season—Late Winter through Spring)

ash	elm	sycamore
birch	hickory	walnut
box elder/maple	mulberry	
cottonwood/poplar	oak	

Grasses (Pollinating Season—Spring through Early Summer)

Bermuda grass	Johnson grass	ryegrass
bluegrass/June grass	orchard grass	Timothy
corn	redtop	

Weeds (Pollinating Season—Summer through Early Fall)

dock/sorrel	Mexican firebush	ragweed—giant,
lamb's quarters	pigweed	short, and western
marsh elder/	plantain	Russian thistle
poverty weed		water hemp

THE GREAT PLAINS

Kansas	North Dakota	South Dakota
Nebraska		

Trees (Pollinating Season—Late Winter through Spring)

alder	cottonwood/poplar	oak
ash	elm	walnut
birch	hazelnut	
box elder/maple	hickory	

Grasses (Pollinating Season—Spring through Early Summer)

bluegrass/June grass	orchard grass	quack grass/wheat
brome	redtop	grass
fescue	ryegrass	Timothy

Weeds (Pollinating Season—Summer through Early Fall)

cocklebur	Mexican firebush	sagebrush
dock/sorrel	pigweed	water hemp
lamb's quarters	plantain	ragweed—false, giant,
marsh elder/poverty weed	Russian thistle	short, and western

SOUTHWESTERN GRASSLANDS

Oklahoma   Texas

Trees (Pollinating Season—Late Winter through Spring)

ash	cottonwood/poplar	mulberry
box elder	elm	oak
cedar/juniper	mesquite	

Grasses (Pollinating Season—Spring through Early Summer)

Bermuda grass	orchard grass	redtop
bluegrass/June grass	quack grass/wheat	ryegrass
fescue	grass	Timothy
Johnson grass		

Weeds (Pollinating Season—Summer through Early Fall)

careless weed/pigweed	marsh elder/poverty	Russian thistle
cocklebur	weed	sagebrush
dock/sorrel	plantain	saltbush/scale
lamb's quarters	ragweed—false, giant,	water hemp
Mexican firebush	short, and western	

ROCKY MOUNTAIN EMPIRE

Arizona (mountainous)	Montana	Wyoming
Colorado	New Mexico	
Idaho (mountainous)	Utah	

Trees (Pollinating Season—Late Winter through Spring)

alder	box elder	elm
ash	cedar/juniper	oak
birch	cottonwood/poplar	pine

Grasses (Pollinating Season—Spring through Early Summer)

Bermuda grass	orchard grass	redtop

bluegrass/June grass	quack grass/wheat	ryegrass
brome	grass	Timothy
fescue		

Weeds (Pollinating Season—Summer through Early Fall)

cocklebur	Mexican firebush	Russian thistle
dock/sorrel	pigweed	sagebrush
lamb's quarters	plantain	saltbush/scale
marsh elder/poverty	ragweed—false, giant,	sugarbeet
weed	short, and western	water hemp

THE ARID SOUTHWEST

Arizona   Southern California (southeast desert)

Trees (Pollinating Season—Winter through Spring)

ash	cypress	olive
cedar/juniper	elm	
cottonwood/poplar	mesquite	

Grasses (Pollinating Season—Spring through Early Summer)

Bermuda grass	brome	ryegrass
bluegrass/June grass	canary grass	salt grass

Weeds (Pollinating Season—Summer through Early Fall)

alkali-blite	lamb's quarters	sagebrush
burro brush	ragweed—false,	saltbush/scale
careless weed	slender, and western	silver ragweed
iodine bush	Russian thistle	

SOUTHERN COASTAL CALIFORNIA

Trees (Pollinating Season—Late Winter through Spring)

acacia	cypress	oak
ash	elm	olive
box elder	eucalyptus	sycamore
cottonwood/poplar	mulberry	walnut

Grasses (Pollinating Season—Spring through Early Summer)

Bermuda grass	fescue	orchard grass
bluegrass/June grass	Johnson grass	ryegrass
brome	oats	salt grass

Weeds (Pollinating Season—Summer through Early Fall)

careless weed/	lamb's quarters	Russian thistle
pigweed	plantain	sagebrush
cocklebur	ragweed—false,	saltbush/scale
dock/sorrel	slender, and western	

THE CENTRAL CALIFORNIA VALLEY

California (Sacramento and San Joaquin valleys)

Trees (Pollinating Season—Late Winter through Spring)

alder	cottonwood/poplar	olive
ash	cypress	pecan
birch	elm	sycamore
box elder	oak	walnut

Grasses (Pollinating Season—Spring through Early Summer)

Bermuda grass	fescue	redtop
bluegrass/June grass	Johnson grass	ryegrass
brome	oats	salt grass
canary grass	orchard grass	Timothy

Weeds (Pollinating Season—Summer through Early Fall)

cocklebur	plantain	sagebrush
dock/sorrel	ragweed—false,	saltbush/scale
lamb's quarters	slender, and western	sugarbeet
pigweed	Russian thistle	

THE INTERMOUNTAIN WEST

Idaho (southern)   Nevada

Trees (Pollinating Season—Late Winter through Spring)

alder	box elder	elm
ash	cedar/juniper	sycamore
birch	cottonwood/poplar	

Grasses (Pollinating Season—Spring through Early Summer)

Bermuda grass	orchard grass	ryegrass
bluegrass/June grass	quack grass/wheat	salt grass
brome	grass	Timothy
fescue	redtop	

Weeds (Pollinating Season—Summer through Early Fall)

cocklebur	Mexican firebush	ragweed—false,
dock/sorrel	pigweed	slender, and
iodine bush	plantain	western
lamb's quarters		Russian thistle
marsh elder/poverty		sagebrush
weed		saltbush/scale

THE INLAND EMPIRE

Oregon (central and   Washington (central
    eastern)   and eastern)

Trees (Pollinating Season—Late Winter through Spring)

alder	cottonwood/poplar	walnut
birch	oak	willow
box elder	pine	

Grasses (Pollinating Season—Spring through Early Summer)

brome	quack grass/	Timothy
bluegrass/June grass	wheatgrass	velvet grass
orchard grass	redtop	vernal grass
	ryegrass	

Weeds (Pollinating Season—Summer through Early Fall)

dock/sorrel	pigweed	ragweed—false, giant,
lamb's quarters	plantain	short, and western
marsh elder/poverty	Russian thistle	
weed	sagebrush	
Mexican firebush	saltbush/scale	

CASCADE PACIFIC NORTHWEST

California	Oregon (western)	Washington (western)
(northwestern)		

Trees (Pollinating Season—Late Winter through Spring)

alder	cottonwood/poplar	walnut
ash	elm	willow
birch	hazelnut	
box elder	oak	

Grasses (Pollinating Season—Spring through Early Summer)

bent grass	fescue	Timothy
Bermuda grass	oats	velvet grass
brome	orchard grass	vernal grass
bluegrass/June grass	ryegrass	
canary grass	salt grass	

Weeds (Pollinating Season—Summer through Early Fall)

cocklebur	plantain	Russian thistle
dock/sorrel	ragweed—false, giant,	sagebrush
lamb's quarters	short, and western	saltbush/scale
pigweed		

ATLANTIC PROVINCES AND QUEBEC

New Brunswick	Nova Scotia	Quebec
Newfoundland	Prince Edward Island	

Trees (Pollinating Season—Late Winter through Spring)

American elm	bur oak	sycamore
balsam poplar	butternut	tag alder

beech	green ash	trembling aspen
black willow	hard maple	white ash
box elder	paper birch	

Grasses (Pollinating Season—Spring through Early Summer)

bluegrass	quack grass	Timothy
brome	redtop	
orchard grass	ryegrass	

Weeds (Pollinating Season—Summer through Early Fall)

| dock/sorrel | plantain | redroot pigweed |
| lamb's quarters | ragweed | Russian thistle |

ONTARIO

Trees (Pollinating Season—Late Winter through Spring)

American elm	box elder	hard maple
aspen	bur oak	paper birch
balsam poplar	butternut	sycamore
beech	Chinese elm	tag alder
black willow	green ash	white ash

Grasses (Pollinating Season—Spring through Early Summer)

bluegrass	quack grass	Timothy
brome	redtop	
orchard grass	ryegrass	

Weeds (Pollinating Season—Summer through Early Fall)

| dock/sorrel | lamb's quarters | redroot pigweed |
| English plantain | ragweed | Russian thistle |

PRAIRIE PROVINCES AND EASTERN BRITISH COLUMBIA

| Alberta | Manitoba | Saskatchewan |
| Eastern British Columbia | | |

Trees (Pollinating Season—Late Winter through Spring)

balsam poplar	Chinese elm	tag alder
box elder	green ash	trembling aspen
bur oak	paper birch	willow

Grasses (Pollinating Season—Spring through Early Summer)

bluegrass	orchard grass	redtop
brome	quack grass (couch)/	ryegrass
common wild oats	wheatgrass	Timothy

Weeds (Pollinating Season—Summer through Early Fall)

| dock/sorrel | marsh elder/poverty | redroot pigweed |

| English plantain | weed | Russian thistle |
| lamb's quarters | ragweed | sagebrush |

WESTERN BRITISH COLUMBIA AND VANCOUVER ISLAND

Trees (Pollinating Season—Late Winter through Spring)

black cottonwood	garry's oak	sycamore
box elder	paper birch	trembling aspen
Chinese elm (Siberian)	red alder	yellow willow
Douglas fir	sitka alder	(Pacific)

Grasses (Pollinating Season—Spring through Early Summer)

bluegrass	orchard grass	ryegrass
brome	quack grass (couch)	tall oat grass
common wild oats	redtop	Timothy

Weeds (Pollinating Season—Summer through Early Fall)

dock/sorrel	marsh elder/poverty	redroot pigweed
English plantain	weed	Russian thistle
lamb's quarters	ragweed	

ALASKA

Trees (Pollinating Season—Spring)

alder	cedar	poplar
aspen	hemlock	spruce
birch	pine	willow

Grasses (Pollinating Season—Late Spring through Summer)

bluegrass/June grass	fescue	redtop
brome	orchard grass	ryegrass
canary grass	quack grass/ wheatgrass	Timothy

Weeds (Pollinating Season—Summer)

bulrush	nettle	sedge
dock/sorrel	plantain	spearscale
lamb's quarters	sagebrush/wormwood	

HAWAII (ALL ISLANDS)

Trees

acacia	date palm	olive
Australian pine (beefwood)	eucalyptus (gum) mesquite	paper mulberry privet
cedar/juniper	Monterey cypress	

Grasses

Bermuda grass	finger grass	redtop
bluegrass/June grass	Johnson grass	sorghum
corn	love grass	

Weeds

cocklebur	plantain	scale (saltbush)
kochia	ragweed, slender	
pigweed	sagebrush	

Note: This was adapted with permission from *Pollen Guide for Allergy*, by Hollister-Stier, 1975.

Appendix C
Moulds Triggering Asthma

Mould	Predominantly Indoor	Predominantly Outdoor
alternaria		X
asperigillus	X	
botrytis		X
curvularia		X
epicocum		X
fusarium		X
geotrichum	X	
helminthosporium		X
hormodendrum		X
mucor		X
nigrospora		X
penicillium	X	
phoma		X
pullularia		X
rhodotorula	X	
stemphylium	X	
streptomyces		X

Appendix D
Food Families

The following two tables show the various food families and the foods found in those families.

Family	Food
apple	apple, crabapple, pear, quince
banana	banana, plantain, psyllium
beech	beechnut, chestnut
birch	filbert, hazelnut
Brazil nut	Brazil nut
buckwheat	buckwheat, garden sorrel, rhubarb
cashew	cashew, mango, pistachio
citrus	grapefruit, kumquat, lemon, lime, orange, tangerine
cola nut	chocolate, cocoa
ebony	persimmon
fungi	mushroom, yeast
ginger	cardamon, ginger, turmeric
gooseberry	currant, gooseberry
goosefoot	beet, spinach, swiss chard
gourd	cantaloupe, cucumber, melon, pumpkin, squash, watermelon, zucchini
grain	bamboo shoots, barley, corn, hominy, malt, oat, rice, rye, sugar cane, wheat
grape	grapes, raisins
heath	blueberry, cranberry, huckleberry
honeysuckle	elderberry

laurel .... avocado, bay leaf, cinnamon, laurel, sassafras

legume .... beans (all types), peas (all types), lentils, licorice, peanuts

lily .... aloes, asparagus, chives, garlic, leek, onion, sarsaparilla, shallot

mallow .... cottonseed, marshmallow, okra

mint .... basil, horehound, marjoram, menthol, mint, oregano, peppermint, rosemary, sage, spearmint, thyme

morning glory .... sweet potato, yam

mulberry .... fig, hops, mulberry

mustard.................... broccoli, Brussels sprout, cabbage, cauliflower, celery, collard, cresses, horseradish, kale, mustard, radish, rutabaga, sauerkraut, turnip

myrtle .... allspice, bayberry, clove, eucalyptus, pimiento

nightshade .... eggplant, pepper (all types except black

.... and white), cayenne, paprika, potato, tabasco, tomato

nutmeg .... mace, nutmeg

olive .... olive (all types)

palm......................... coconut, date, palm oil

parsley...................... anise, caraway, carrot, celery, coriander, cumin, dill, fennel, parsley, parsnips, water celery

pepper...................... black and white pepper only

pineapple.................. pineapple

plum .... almond, apricot, cherry, nectarine, peach, plum, prune

rose .... blackberry, blackthorn, dewberry, loganberry, raspberry

sunflower .... chickory, endive, lettuce, sunflower seed, tarra-
(composite) .... gon, yarrow

walnut .... butternut, hickory nut, pecan, walnut

Animal Family	Food
amphibians	frog
birds........................	chicken, duck, goose, pheasant, quail, turkey
crustaceans	crab, crayfish, lobster, prawn, shrimp
eggs	various bird eggs
mammals..................	cow, goat, lamb, pig, pork, rabbit, sheep, squirrel

milk products .... butter, cheese, cream, milk, yogurt

mollusks .... abalone, clam, cockle, mussel, octopus, oyster, scallop, snail, squid

reptiles .... alligator, crocodile, snake, turtle

---

Note: Sometimes heating in the preparation of food will denature the allergic protein. Thus, eating the cooked food won't cause an allergic reaction even though there's a positive reaction on testing.

Appendix E
Asthma Breathing Aids, and How To Use Them

Hand-Held Inhalers

Hand-held inhalers propel asthma medication into the lungs. There are several devices manufactured by various companies, and they all function similarly.

When using these inhalers, timing is important to get the medicine into the lungs. It is important to simultaneously compress the inhaler to release the medicine while you are inhaling.

For proper use:

- make sure the drug canister is properly inserted into the inhaler,
- shake the inhaler before use,
- place the inhaler into your mouth and breathe out normally,
- breathe in slowly and deeply while pressing the canister down firmly to release the flow of medication to the lungs,
- hold your breath for 5 to 10 seconds after inhaling the medicine to allow it to spread throughout your lungs,
- keep the cap on the inhaler when you're not using it—and clean the inhaler frequently with plain water and wipe it dry, and
- do not take the medicine more frequently than prescribed.

Sometimes it's difficult to achieve the proper technique. To be sure you are using the inhaler properly, stand in front of a mirror, compress the inhaler when you start a deep breath, and hold your breath for 5 seconds before exhaling. If you see fog coming out of your mouth while inhaling or exhaling, the medication hasn't reached your lungs. If you don't see fog, you've used the inhaler properly.

Adaptors for Hand-Held Inhalers

There are adaptors for hand-held inhalers that eliminate the need of timing your inhalation with your compression of the inhaler. These devices consist of a chamber that catches the propelled mist from the inhaler and holds it until a full, deep inhalation can carry it to your lungs.

Adaptors are especially helpful for young children and others who have difficulty learning the proper technique for using hand-held inhalers.

Adaptors can be found under the following trade names: Inhal-Aid, Inspirease, Aero-Chamber, and Brethancer.

Another type of adaptor, especially designed for arthritics having difficulty compressing hand-held inhalers, is what's called a Vent Ease. This device delivers medication by a simple flick of the finger, and is easy to use for anyone with hand-movement problems.

Spinhalers

This device propels cromolyn sodium powder into the lungs. The powder comes in a capsule, which you load into the Spinhaler. Then the capsule is pierced by moving the outer covering up and down. The powder is propelled into the lungs when a deep inhalation causes an inner propeller to spin.

Motorized Nebulizers and Intermittent Positive Pressure Breathing (IPPB) Machines

Both types of machines generate an asthma-medication mist that is inhaled into the lungs, and both provide quick optimal delivery of medication to the lungs. They are most helpful for acute attacks and are rarely necessary on a regular basis. Although they are most commonly used in doctor's offices and emergency rooms, they can be used at home if needed. They're very helpful for people who get severe and frequent asthma attacks because they can provide rapid relief. People living far from medical facilities find these devices very convenient—especially in the middle of the night.

The medicine dose is diluted in salt water (1 teaspoon salt/1 quart of water) and placed in a reservoir on the machine. When the machine starts, it turns the solution into a mist that is easily inhaled into the lungs.

Appendix F
Asthma Day or Resident Camps for Children in the United States

Day Camps for Children with Asthma

Arizona Lung Association
102 West McDowell Road
Phoenix, Arizona 85003

ALA of Alameda County
295 27th Street
Oakland, California 94612

ALA of Contra Costa-Solano
105 Astrid Drive
Pleasant Hill, California 90813

Long Beach Lung Association
1002 Pacific Avenue
Long Beach, California 94523

ALA of Monterey, Santa Cruz
& San Luis Obispo Counties
140 Central Avenue
Salinas, California 93901

ALA of Riverside County
3600 Lime Street—Suite 415
Riverside, California 92501

ALA of San Bernardino, Inyo &
Mono Counties
371 West 14th Street
San Bernardino, California 92405

ALA of San Francisco
833 Market Street—9th Floor
San Francisco, California 94103

ALA of San Mateo County
2250 Palm Avenue
San Mateo, California 94403

ALA of Santa Clara-San Benito
Counties
1469 Park Avenue
San Jose, California 95126

ALA of Superior California
2720 Cohasset Road #B
Chico, California 95926

ALA of Central Florida
2737 Fern Creek
Orlando, Florida 32806

Illinois Valley Lung Assn.
2126 North Sheridan Road
Peoria, Illinois 61604

ALA of North Central Indiana
6685 Broadway
Merrilleville, Indiana 46410

ALA of Northwest Indiana
442½ Fifth Street
Columbus, Indiana 47201

ALA of Genesee Valley
1511 West Third Avenue
Flint, Michigan 48504

ALA of Nevada
75 Kirman Avenue
Reno, Nevada 89502

New Hampshire Lung Assn.
456 Beech Street
Manchester, New Hampshire
03103

ALA of Nassau-Suffolk
405 Ostrander Avenue
Riverhead, New York 11901

ALA of Ohio
Eastern Central Branch
1036 Wheeling Avenue
Cambridge, Ohio 43725

Asociacion Puertorriquena del
Pulmon
395 Domenech Avenue
Hato Rey, Puerto Rico 00918

ALA of South Carolina
1817 Gadsden Street
Columbia, South Carolina 29201

Day Camps for Children with Asthma in Cooperation with Others

ALA of Monterey, Santa Cruz &
San Luis Obispo Counties
140 Central Avenue
Salinas, California 93901

ALA of Riverside County
3600 Lime Street—Suite 415
Riverside, California 92501

ALA of Central Florida
2737 Fern Creek Avenue
Orlando, Florida 32806

ALA of San Bernardino, Inyo &
Mono Counties
371 West 14th Street
San Bernardino, California 92405

ALA of Hawaii
245 North Kukui Street
Honolulu, Hawaii 96817

Illinois Valley Lung Association
2126 North Sheridan Road
Peoria, Illinois 61604

ALA of North Central Indiana
319 South Main Street
South Bend, Indiana 46601

ALA of Genesee Valley
1511 West Third Avenue
Flint, Michigan 48504

ALA of Western Massachusetts
393 Maple Street
Springfield, Massachusetts 01105

Resident Camps for Children with Asthma

Alaska Lung Association
406 "G" Street
Anchorage, Alaska 99501

ALA of Arkansas
412 West Seventh Street
Little Rock, Arkansas 72201

ALA of Central California
234 North Broadway
Fresno, California 93701

ALA of Los Angeles County
5858 Wilshire Blvd—Suite 300
Los Angeles, California 90036

ALA of Orange County
1717 North Broadway
Santa Ana, California 92706

Pasadena Lung Association
111 North Hudson Avenue
Pasadena, California 91101

ALA of San Bernardino, Inyo &
Mono Counties
371 West 14th Street
San Bernardino, California 92405

ALA of San Diego & Imperial
Counties
3861 Front Street
San Diego, California 92103

ALA of Santa Clara-San Benito
Counties
1469 Park Avenue
San Jose, California 95126

ALA of Ventura County
1767 East Main Street
Ventura, California 93001

ALA of Colorado
1600 Race Street
Denver, Colorado 80206

ALA of Florida
5526 Arlington Road
Jacksonville, Florida 32211

ALA of Florida/Spaceport
Branch
412 South Palmetto Avenue
Daytona Beach, Florida 32014

ALA of Broward-Glades-Hendry
2020 South Andrews Avenue
Ft. Lauderdale, Florida 33316

ALA of Central Florida
2737 Fern Creek
Orlando, Florida 32806

ALA of Dade-Monroe
830 Brickell Plaza
Miami, Florida 33131

Gulf Coast Lung Association
6160 Central Avenue
St. Petersburg, Florida 33707

ALA of Southwest Florida
2300 Euclid Avenue
Ft. Myers, Florida 33901

ALA of Atlanta
723 Piedmont Avenue, NE
Atlanta, Georgia 30365

Chicago Lung Association
1440 W. Washington Boulevard
Chicago, IL 60607

ALA of Illinois
One Christmas Seal Drive
725 South 26th Street
Springfield, IL 62703

ALA of DuPage & McHenry
Counties
526 Crescent Blvd.—Room 216
Glen Ellyn, Illinois 60137

Illinois Valley Lung Association
2126 North Sheridan Road
Peoria, Illinois 61604

Lake Country Lung Association
813 Washington Street
Waukegan, Illinois 61764

ALA of Mid-Eastern Illinois
110 West Water Street—Suite
B-4
Pontiac, Illinois 61764

ALA of Central Indiana
615 North Alabama Street—
Room 335
Indianapolis, Indiana 46204

ALA of Northeast Indiana
802 West Wayne Street
Ft. Wayne, Indiana 46804

ALA of Southeast Indiana
$442\frac{1}{2}$ Fifth Street
Columbus, Indiana 47201

ALA of Southwest Indiana
Seven East Columbia Street
Evansville, Indiana 47711

ALA of Iowa
1321 Walnut Street
Des Moines, Iowa 50309

ALA of Kansas
4300 Drury Lane
Topeka, Kansas 66604

ALA of Boston
263 Summer Street
Boston, Massachusetts 02210

ALA of Central Massachusetts
35 Harvard Street
Worcester, Massachusetts 01609

ALA of Essex County
239 Newburyport Turnpike/
Route #1
Topsfield, Massachusetts 01983

ALA of Middlesex County
Five Mountain Road
Burlington, Massachusetts 01803

Norfolk County-Newton Lung
Assn.
25 Spring Street
Walpole, Massachusetts 02081

ALA of Southeastern Massachusetts
West Grove Street/Route 28
Middleboro, Massachusetts
02346

ALA of Western Massachusetts
393 Maple Street
Springfield, Massachusetts 01105

ALA of Central New Jersey
206 Westfield Avenue
Clark, New Jersey 07066

ALA of New Mexico
216 Truman NE
Albuquerque, New Mexico
87108

ALA of Mid-New York
23 South Street
Utica, New York 13501

ALA of North Dakota
212 North Second Street
Bismarck, North Dakota 58501

ALA of Southeastern Michigan
28 West Adams Street
Detroit, Michigan 48226

ALA of Michigan
403 Seymour Avenue
Lansing, Michigan 48914

ALA of Hennepin County
1829 Portland Avenue
Minneapolis, Minnesota 55404

ALA of Ramsey County
614 Portland Avenue
St. Paul, Minnesota 55102

ALA of Eastern Missouri
1118 Hampton Avenue
St. Louis, Missouri 63139

ALA of Montana
825 Helena Avenue
Helena, Montana 59601

ALA of Nebraska
8901 Indian Hills Dr.—Suite
107
Omaha, Nebraska 68114

New Hampshire Lung Association
456 Beech Street
Manchester, New Hampshire
03103

ALA of Ohio
1700 Arlingate Lane
Columbus, Ohio 43228

ALA of Ohio/East Central
Branch
1036 Wheeling Avenue
Cambridge, Ohio 43725

ALA of Ohio/North Central
Branch
200 Newark Road—Suite B
Mt. Vernon, Ohio 43050

ALA of Ohio/South East Branch
527-B Richland Avenue
Athens, Ohio 45701

ALA of Ohio/South Shore
Branch
16 West Church Street
Milan, Ohio 44846

ALA of Ohio/Summit County
Branch
1772 State Road—2nd Floor
Cuyahoga Falls, Ohio 44223

ALA of Ohio/Western Branch
1034 West Market Street
Lima, Ohio 45805

ALA of Northern Ohio
4614 Prospect Avenue—Room 307
Cleveland, Ohio 44103

ALA of Northwestern Ohio
520 Madison Avenue—Suite 225
Toledo, Ohio 43604

ALA of Southwestern Ohio
2330 Victory Parkway
Cincinnati, Ohio 45206

ALA of Stark-Wayne
1300 Christmas Seal Drive NW
Canton, Ohio 44709

ALA of Oklahoma
2442 North Walnut
Oklahoma City, Oklahoma 73105

ALA of Green Country Oklahoma
5553 South Peoria
Tulsa, Oklahoma 74105

Oregon Lung Association
319 SW Washington St.—Suite 520
Portland, Oregon 97204

ALA of Delaware/Chester Counties
1502 West Chester Pike
West Chester, Pennsylvania 19382

ALA of Northeast Pennsylvania
302 North Main Avenue
Scranton, Pennsylvania 18504

ALA of Northwest Pennsylvania
352 West Eighth Street
Erie, Pennsylvania 16502

ALA of Southwestern Pennsylvania
409 South Main Street
Greensburg, Pennsylvania 15601

Asociacion Puertorriquena Del Pulmon
395 Domenech Avenue
Hato Rey, Puerto Rico 00918

ALA of South Carolina
1817 Gadsden Street
Columbia, South Carolina 29201

ALA of Utah
1930 South 1100 East
Salt Lake City, Utah 84106

ALA of Wisconsin
10001 West Lisbon Avenue
Milwaukee, Wisconsin 53222

Note: The American Lung Association provided this list.

Appendix G
Products For Treating Allergy, and Where To Find Them

HEPA Filters

Airstar-5
AllerMed Corporation
PO Box 865769 (APD)
Plano, TX 75086
214–248–0782
Portable HEPA; charcoal, formaldehyde filters

Air Techniques, Inc.
1801 Whitehead Road (APD)
Baltimore, MD 21207
301–944–6037
Furnace, room-size HEPA filters with charcoal pre- and post-filters

Bio Medisphere
565 Commerce Street (APD)
Franklin Lakes, NJ 07417
1–800–222–0577
HEPA filter

Cleanaire HEPA
Bio-Tech Systems
PO Box 25380 (APD)
Chicago, IL 60625
1–800–621–5545
Furnace, room-size HEPA filters

Control Resource Systems, Inc.
670 Mariner Drive (APD)
PO Box 421 (APD)
Michigan City, IN 46360
HEPA air filtration units

ExcelAir
HMD, Inc. (APD)
Birmingham, MI
313–645–6707
HEPA-filtered air flows through bed headboard.

Hepanaire Air Cleaner
Summit Hill Laboratories
429 Highway 36 (APD)
PO Box 535 (APD)
Navesink, NJ 07752
1-800-922-0722
Portable HEPA filter

Electrostatic Precipitators

Electrostatic Air Filter
Hi-Tech Filter Corporation of
America
80 Myrtle Street (APD)
North Quincy, MA 02171
1-800-448-3249
Replaces furnace and air-conditioner filters; washable, reusable; also as HEPA prefilter.

Honeywell Clean Air Machine
Honeywell
Honeywell Plaza
Minneapolis, MN 55408
Electronic air cleaner

Micronaire Air Cleaner
Summit Hill Laboratories
429 Highway 36 (APD)
PO Box 535 (APD)
Navesink, NJ 07752
1-800-922-0722
Portable, electrostatic air filter

Newtron Electrostatic Air
Cleaner
Newtron Products Company
3874 Virginia Avenue (APD)
PO Box 27175 (APD)
Cincinnati, OH 45227-0175
1-800-543-9149
Replaces present filter in heating and air-conditioning systems.

Sanitron Electronic Air Cleaner
Duralast Products Corporation
PO Box 15869 (APD)
New Orleans, LA 70175

Vietech Electrostatic Air Cleaner
Vietech Limited
10 Gore Street (APD)
London, Ontario
Canada N5W 4A7
519-451-2694
Nonelectronic electrostatic air cleaner

You may find local distributors of air cleaners under "Air Conditioning" in the telephone directory.

Mattress and Pillow Enclosures

Allergen-Proof Encasings
1450 East 363rd Street (APD)
Eastlake, OH 44094
216–946–6700

Allergy Control Products
28 High Ridge Road (APD)
Ridgefield, CT 06877

Bio-Tech Systems
Post Office Box 25380 (APD)
Chicago, IL 60625
1–800–621–5545
in Illinois 312–465–8020

Aller Guard
Medical Plaza Building
Post Office Box 58027 (APD)
Topeka, KS 66658

Environtrol Aller-Shield
Environtrol Corporation
PO Box 31313 (APD)
St. Louis, MO 63131
1–800–423–1982
in Missouri: 314–966–6686

Micro Filtration Limited
42 Hardwick Industrial Estate
Bury St. Edmunds
Suffolk, United Kingdom
1P33 2QLHH

Dehumidifiers

Check local department stores or
these national distributors:
  Comfort Air
  Fedders
  Kelvinator
  Oasis

General Allergy Products Information

Write to: The Allergy Products
Directory
  P.O. Box 640
  Menlo Park, CA 94026

Mould Control Chemicals

Allergen-Proof Encasings, Inc.
1450 East 363rd St.
Eastlake, OH 44094
(216) 946-6700
    A.P.E. Mold Remover
    A.P.E. 100 Mold Remover
    and Preventative
    Greer Disinfectant Deodorant
    Impregon

Bio-Tech Systems
PO Box 25380
Chicago, IL 60625
(800) 621-5545; in Illinois
(312) 465-8020
    R.E.P. 10 Mold Remover
    R.E.P. 60 Mold Preventer

Glossary

Adrenal gland   An organ just above the kidney that manufactures steroids. It's the only source of adrenocorticosteroids in our body.

Adrenocorticosteroids Steroids produced by the adrenal gland that help our organs and tissues adapt to a constantly changing environment and allow our bodies to perform with relative freedom. Drugs similar to adrenocorticosteroids are used in the treatment of asthma.

Allergen   Also called antigen, this is any substance that can cause an allergic reaction.

Allergic reaction   A reaction caused by an allergy that results in adverse symptoms. This term encompasses many different types of adverse reactions caused by many different allergens. The type of reaction depends on the allergen substance, how it gets into the body, and the allergic person's immunologic response (what type of antibody is formed or cell is activated to attack the allergen).

Allergic rhinitis   An allergy-triggered nasal condition, often referred to as hay fever.

Allergist   A physician who specializes in the diagnosis and treatment of allergies and asthma.

Allergy   A condition caused by the immune system overreacting, leaving a person hypersensitive to a substance (allergen) that is normally harmless to the general population.

Allergy season   Any time of the year in which there is a heavy load of any particular type of allergen (for example, ragweed-pollen season in late summer and early fall in the midwestern United States).

Allergy shots   *See* Immunotherapy.

Alpha-1 antitrypsin   An enzyme that protects the lungs from the development of emphysema. A lack of this enzyme may result in early emphysema. A blood test can be used to test for this enzyme.

Aminophylline   A theophyllinelike drug used in the treatment of asthma.

Antibiotics   Drugs used to treat bacterial infections.

Antibodies   A specifically structured protein found in the blood and body fluids produced by the immune system in response to a foreign invader, such as a virus, bacteria, cancerous growth, allergen, or organ transplant. It is referred to chemically as an immunoglobulin. It generally falls into one of five classes (IgG, IgA, IgM, IgD, and IgE), each of which performs a different immune defense job. IgE, through its defensive action, causes allergic symptoms, such as extrinsic asthma.

Antigen   Any foreign substance that produces an immune reaction. An antigen is referred to as an allergen when it produces an immune reaction that results in allergic symptoms.

Antihistamines   Drugs used to treat allergy and cold symptoms of the nose. They work by blocking histamine and drying secretions.

Arterial blood gases   A test to measure the concentration of the two major gases carried by our arterial blood. They can be an accurate measurement of the severity of asthma and other pulmonary diseases.

Asthma   A condition of a supersensitive state of the windpipes, resulting in airway obstruction when stimulated by various triggers. The obstruction can vary in degree and duration, and is partially or completely reversible, either spontaneously or after treatment.

Asthma, classifications of:

Mild asthma   Less than six mild attacks per year; minimal or no symptoms between attacks; normal functioning between attacks; requires little or no medication between attacks; causes no loss of school or work; and requires no hospitalizations.

Moderate asthma   More than six moderate attacks per year; mild symptoms between attacks; mild functional impairment between attacks; often requires medication between attacks; causes loss of up to 10 days of school or work per year; and requires one or no hospitalization(s) per year.

Severe asthma   More than six severe attacks per year, despite continued medication; mild to moderate symptoms between attacks; moderate to severe functional impairment between attacks; causes loss of more than 10 days of school or work per year; and requires two or more hospitalizations per year.

Atelectasis   The collapse of a lung segment from mucous plugging and narrowing of a windpipe during asthma.

Atopic dermatitis (eczema)   Inflammatory disease of the skin associated with allergies. Usual locations are behind the knees and in front of the elbows. It is often associated with dry skin all over the body.

Atopy   The capacity to develop immediate sensitivity (allergy) to common allergens upon natural exposure, demonstrated by skin tests and mediated by IgE antibody.

Autonomic nervous system The part of the nervous system that is not under a person's voluntary control. It regulates the function of many organ systems in our body, including the respiratory system.

Beta stimulators A group of drugs used in the treatment of asthma that dilate the windpipes by stimulating the beta-adrenergic nervous system, which, when activated, dilates the bronchial tubes.

Biofeedback A procedure involving use of a measuring device for muscle tension or skin temperature change to assist in determining a tense or truly relaxed state. This is very helpful in stress reduction when used with other relaxation techniques.

Bronchial provocation test A kind of pulmonary function test that provokes the bronchial tubes into spasm in an asthmatic. It can be used to diagnose asthma when an attack is not present. (*See* Methacholine pulmonary function test.)

Bronchial tubes Airway tubes, or windpipes, that bring air from the trachea to the alveoli (tiny air sacs in the lungs where oxygen is transferred to the blood).

Bronchitis A lung disease due to inflammation of the bronchial mucous membranes resulting in increased mucous production. Most commonly due to cigarette smoking, but other environmental substances may play a role. In children it is usually caused by a virus.

Bronchodilator A generic term for any drug that can dilate the bronchial tubes.

Bronchospasm A narrowing of airways that occurs during an asthma attack.

Carbon dioxide Abbreviated as CO_2, this gas is the waste product from our tissues that is picked up by our blood and delivered to our lungs for removal during breathing.

Chronic obstructive pulmonary disease Abbreviated as COPD, it includes several major respiratory diseases, such as bronchitis, emphysema, and asthma.

Cromolyn sodium A medication taken by inhalation that is used to prevent and control asthma. It is most effective in treating extrinsic asthma and asthma triggered by exercise. It works by inhibiting the release of mediators of asthma.

Cyanosis A bluish discoloration of the lips and the nails occurring when the blood oxygen level is low.

Diaphragm A large muscle between the chest and abdomen that works as a bellows for the lungs as it moves down into the abdomen. During inhalation, it enlarges the chest cavity, and the lungs expand, filling with air. It moves into the chest cavity during exhalation and forces air out of the lungs.

Diaphragmatic breathing Known as "belly breathing" or relaxed breathing, this is the correct way of breathing for everyone and promotes a relaxed state. When properly done, the abdomen moves out as the diaphragm moves down during inhalation; the reverse occurs during exhalation.

Dust mite A minuscule living organism found in house dust, especially mattress dust, which feeds on human skin particles. It is a major allergen in house dust.

Eczema Also known as dermatitis or an inflammation of the skin. In this book, it refers specifically to atopic eczema or atopic dermatitis (inflammatory disease of the skin associated with allergies). (*See* Atopic dermatitis.)

Electrostatic precipitator A special filter effective in removing dust, allergens, and irritants from the environment by use of electrically charged plates. Suitable for stand-alone portable units and for attachment to central heating units.

Emphysema A lung disease resulting in destruction of air sacs, usually caused by cigarette smoking in susceptible individuals.

Environmental control Avoidance measures used to minimize exposure to allergens and other triggers for asthma in the environment.

Eosinophil A type of white blood cell often elevated in the blood, sputum, and nasal secretions in allergic conditions and certain nonallergic conditions, such as intrinsic asthma.

Eustachian tubes Tubes leading from behind the nose to the middle ear that are important for getting air into the middle ear for proper functioning of the eardrums.

Exercise-induced asthma (EIA) Asthma triggered by physical exertion, especially running, particularly in cold, dry air.

Extrinsic asthma Asthma that is generally triggered by allergic factors or allergens. This is also known as allergic asthma or atopic asthma.

Forced expiratory volume in 1 second (FEV_1) A measurement of the maximum *speed* of air movement out of the lungs during exhalation. Actually, a measurement of the volume of exhaled air during the first second of forced exhalation.

Forced vital capacity (FVC) A measurement of the maximum *amount* of air moved out of the lungs during total exhalation.

HEPA filters High-efficiency particulate air filters effective in removing many allergens and irritants from the inside environment, and generally used as a stand-alone portable unit.

Histamine   The most well known—but not necessarily the most important—chemical mediator in allergic reactions. It is stored in mast cells in our body.

Hyperventilation   Over-breathing by increasing the rate of breathing and/or increasing the volume of air in each breath. Either way, too much carbon dioxide is "blown off," resulting in a low CO_2 level in the blood, which causes several adverse symptoms.

IgE antibody   A class of antibody that, although the least abundant, is the most important in causing allergic reactions, including extrinsic asthma and allergic rhinitis. It concentrates in the lining of the respiratory system, in the gastrointestinal system, and in the skin by attaching to mast cells located in these areas.

Immune system   The system in the body responsible for protection against foreign invaders, such as bacteria, viruses, cancer growths, and other substances. It performs its job in part by producing antibodies to attack and destroy foreign invaders.

Immunoglobulins   Proteins in the blood that form antibodies that are important in defense against invading viruses, bacteria, and parasites. They also are responsible for many allergic reactions. There are five major immunoglobulin classes: IgG, IgA, IgM, IgD, and IgE (*see* Antibodies).

Immunology   The study of the immune system in its relationship to health and disease.

Immunotherapy (allergy shots)   A method of injecting an individual with small but increasing doses of a substance to which he is allergic, with the intent to beneficially alter his immune or allergic response.

Intradermal skin test   A kind of allergy skin test where an injection of a tiny amount of allergen is placed just under the skin.

Intrinsic asthma   Asthma that is generally triggered by nonallergic factors and due to an intrinsic, supersensitive condition of the windpipes.

Mast cells   Cells containing chemical mediators that are found throughout the body, but more so in areas exposed to the environment, such as the skin and the mucous membrane of the respiratory tract and GI tract. They release their chemical mediators during allergic reactions, which causes changes in the body (*see* IgE antibody).

Mediators   Chemicals released from mast cells that cause bronchospasm or inflammation of bronchi in an asthmatic. They are usually released during an allergic reaction, but other phenomena may cause their release.

Meditation   A technique used for inducing relaxation by training the mind to concentrate on a simple phrase or word (known as a mantra), which, in turn, helps to block out stressful thoughts.

Methacholine pulmonary function test   A type of pulmonary function test that measures a person's volume (vital capacity) and flow of air (forced expiratory volume in one second) before and after inhalation of a measured dose of methacholine. It is commonly used in the diagnosis of asthma by showing a decrease in a person's volume and flow of air after inhaling methacholine.

Morbidity   The characteristics of a disease that interfere with an individual's ability to function normally.

Mortality   The term applied to the rate or numbers of deaths from a disease.

Mould   A low class of plant without chlorophyll that must live off other dead or living organic matter and reproduce by expelling large numbers of spores into the air. Mould is a common cause of allergy.

Nasal polyps   A protruding growth of the mucous membrane of the nose or sinus resulting in obstruction. It can be associated with asthma as well as other conditions.

Nebulizer   A device that converts a liquid into a fine spray for inhalation.

Nonsteroidal anti-inflammatory drugs (NSAID)   Potent drugs that work much like aspirin to inhibit inflammation and pain. These drugs include:

•ibuprofen (Motrin, Advil, Nuprin, Ibuprin, Mediprin, Pamprin-IB, Haltran, Expain, and others),

•naproxen (Naprosyn and Anaprox),

•fenoprofen (Nalfon),

•meclofenamate (Meclomen),

•piroxicam (Feldene),

•sulindac (Clinoril),

•tolmetin (Tolectin),

•ketoprofen (Orudis),

•indomethacin (Indocin),

•phenylbutazone (Butazolidin), and

•diflunisal (Dolobid).

Occupational asthma   Asthma caused from the workplace environment.

Parasympathetic nervous system   Also known as the cholinergic nervous system, this is a part of the autonomic nervous system that increases the tone of smooth muscle (resulting in windpipe contraction) and increases secretions.

Pneumomediastinum   The development of air in the tissue between the lungs due to leaking of air from ruptured air sacs in the lungs.

Pneumonia   A lung infection caused by a virus or bacteria.

Pneumothorax   The development of air between the outer surface of the lung and the chest wall, causing partial or total collapse of the lung.

Pollen   The living male germinal cells in plants—such as trees, grasses, and weeds—needed for fertilization and reproduction. These cells are tiny seedlike grains, which range in microscopic sizes and are transported to other plants by insects and the wind. Wind-transported pollens (aeroallergens) are a common cause of allergy.

Pollen count   An indirect measurement of the amount of pollen in the air.

Pollination   The act of shedding pollen that occurs at different times of the year for different species of plants.

Prednisone   A common steroid drug used in the treatment of asthma (*see* Steroids).

Progressive muscle relaxation   A self-help relaxation technique whereby individual muscle groups are alternately tensed and relaxed to promote a totally relaxed body state.

Psychosomatic   Physical symptoms resulting from emotional or stressful situations.

Pulmonary function test   A method of determining the capacity and function of the lungs. This is done by use of a spirometer, which measures a person's volume and flow of exhaled air. It's recorded as vital capacity (VC) and forced expiratory volume in one second (FEV_1).

RAST test (Radioallergosorbent test)   A sophisticated blood test that measures the small quantity of allergic antibodies (IgE antibodies) in the blood that will react with a specific allergen.

Reflex bronchospasm   The stimulation of airway irritant receptors that cause a reflex increased activity of the vagus nerve, resulting in bronchospasm.

Relaxed breathing   *See* Diaphragmatic breathing.

Scratch test   A kind of allergy skin test where allergens are applied to tiny scratches that penetrate only the top layer of skin.

Sinusitis   An inflammation of the sinuses, usually caused by a bacterial infection although allergy or other conditions may play a significant role.

Skin tests   Tests to determine the presence of allergy by placing a small amount of test allergen on or just under the skin. There are two types of skin tests: scratch and intradermal.

Somatopsychic   Emotional or stress symptoms resulting from a physical illness.

Status asthmaticus   Asthma out of control that doesn't readily respond to medical treatment. It usually requires hospitalization and can be life-threatening.

Steroids (adrenocorticosteroids)   Powerful agents that have an action similar to that of the hormones released from the adrenal glands, and are commonly used in the treatment of asthma and many other diseases.

Stress   Your body's response—positive or negative—to any demand (stressor) made on it. It involves a response through the autonomic nervous system, resulting in multiple emotional and physical symptoms.

Stress breathing   Rapid, shallow breathing mainly with the use of the upper-chest muscles, which may stimulate the sympathetic nervous system to produce a widespread stress response.

Stressor   Events or circumstances that cause the stress response.

Sulfites   Food preservatives that are a known cause for asthma symptoms in some asthmatics. They cause asthma through mechanisms other than allergy.

Sweat chloride test   A measurement of the sweat for chloride. It is significantly elevated in individuals with cystic fibrosis.

Sympathetic nervous system   Also known as the adrenergic nervous system, this is a part of the autonomic nervous system that decreases the tone of smooth muscle (resulting in windpipe dilatation) and decreases secretions.

Tartrazine (FD&C Yellow #5)   A yellow dye commonly used to color foods and drugs that is incriminated as a trigger for asthma (controversial).

Theophylline   A powerful bronchodilator closely related chemically to caffeine and commonly used in the treatment of asthma. It acts directly on the muscles of the airways to relax and open them.

Trigger   A substance or condition, internal or external, that can induce an asthma attack.

Vasomotor rhinitis   An inflammation of the nose that occurs because of an increased sensitivity of the nasal membrane to irritating substances, viral infections, weather changes, and stress.

Visualization   A technique that is used to help induce relaxation by visualizing, or picturing, a relaxed image in the mind.

Wheeze   A high-pitched sound made by air passing through windpipes that are narrowed during an asthma attack. It is usually heard upon expiration.

About the Authors

Glennon H. Paul is a graduate of the St. Louis College of Pharmacy and the University of Missouri School of Medicine. He did postdoctoral training in Internal Medicine and Allergy at the University of Washington in Seattle. Now based in Springfield, Illinois, Dr. Paul is the medical director of respiratory therapy at St. John's Hospital and a clinical assistant professor of medicine at the Southern Illinois University School of Medicine, and also is in private practice. He is a fellow of both the American Academy of Allergy and the American College of Chest Physicians.

Barbara A. Fafoglia is an English-teacher-turned-writer, who works in Springfield, Illinois, as a communications specialist for a drug-and-alcohol-abuse prevention center and as a consulting writer and editor for Southern Illinois University School of Medicine.

Index

Index

A

Absenteeism, 147–148
Acetylsalicylic acid (aspirin), 37, 99
Acid anhydrides, 166
Acne, from steroids, 96
Activity, physical, childhood asthma and, 53
Acute asthma, short-acting theophylline preparations for, 104
Acute epiglottis, 52
Adaptors, for hand-held inhalers, 104
Adenoids, 63
Adrenal gland, 223
    suppression, from steroids, 95, 98
Adrenaline. *See* Epinephrine
Adrenocorticosteroids. *See* Steroids
Adult asthma, vs. childhood asthma, 44–45
Aeroallergens, 22
Aerobid, 101
Aero-Chamber, 104
Age, 14
    effect on skin testing, 64
    of onset, 72
        for intrinsic asthma, 35, 36
    risk of death and, 143

Airflow obstruction, 69–70
Air pollution, 41–42
Airways
    obstruction of, in differential diagnosis of lung disease, 69–70
    twitchy or hyperactive, 15, 35–36, 44
Albuterol (salbutamol)
    effects on mother and fetus, 129
    inhaled, 84
    oral, 85
Alcalase, 170
Alcohol
    effects on beta stimulators, 88
    effects on cromolyn, 89
    effects on steroids, 100
    effects on theophylline, 80
Alder pollen, 23
Allergens, 19, 20, 223
    in classroom, 152
    inhaled, status asthmaticus development and, 135
    miscellaneous, 32
    suitable for environmental control, 110–113
    triggering extrinsic asthma, 21–34
Allergic asthma. *See* Extrinsic asthma

Allergic reactions, 20, 223
  from occupational asthma,
    164–165
Allergic rhinitis, 223
Allergic salute, 62
Allergic shiners, 62
Allergist, 223
  advantages in consulting, 58
  first visit, 60–67
  preparation for first visit, 58–59
Allergy, 17–18, 223
  characteristics of, 19
  precautions to decrease incidence
    or delay in development in
    infant, 132
Allergy season, 223
Allergy shots. See Immunotherapy
Alpha-amylase, 170
Alpha-1 antitrypsin, 223
  test for, 66
Alupent, 83, 84, 85
Alveoli, 192
Aminoethylethanolamine, 168
Aminophylline, 140, 223
Ammonium thioglycolate, 168
Ampicillin, usage during pregnancy,
    130
Analgesics, 37
Androgenic steroids, 90
Anesthesia
  effect on asthma, 121–122
  options for asthmatics, 121
Anesthetic-inducing agents, 122
Anger, childhood asthma and, 54
Animals
  causing occupational asthma,
    170–171
  consideration as trigger, 61
  dander from, 31
    environmental control measures,
      112
Antiallergic mediator agents, 76
Antibiotics, 140, 224
  beneficial use in asthmatics, 107
  effects on mother and fetus, 130

troleandomycin, use with
    methylprednisolone, 106
Antibodies, 20, 224
  blocking, 115
Anticholinergic drugs, 108
Antigen, 223, 224. See also Allergens
Antihistamines, 107, 116, 224
  effects on mother and fetus,
    129–130
  skin testing and, 64
Anti-inflammatory agents, 76
Appetite, steroids and, 93
Aprolium hydrochloride,
    occupational asthma from, 169
Aristocort, 94
Arterial blood gases, 224
Artificial ventilation, 141
Asbestosis, 175
Aseptic bone necrosis, 97
Ash pollen, 23
Aspirated objects, 51
Aspirin
  sensitivity to, 37
  steroids and, 99
Asthma. See also specific aspects of
  basic facts about, 14–18
  characteristics of, 15
  definition of, 224
  differential diagnosis, 68–70
    differences from bronchitis and
      emphysema, 72–73
    by doctor, 70–71
Asthma attacks
  anesthesia and, 119
  characteristics of, 15–16
  out of control, indicators for,
    136–137
  severity of, 16–17
  surgery and, 119
  time of, mortality risk and,
    142–143
  triggers for, 17
Asthma triad, 37
Atelectasis, 123, 138, 141, 224
Atopic dermatitis, 37, 224

Atopy
    definition of, 224–225
    occupational asthma and, 163
Atrovent (ipratropium bromide), 108
Autonomic nervous system, 225
Avoidance measures. *See*
    Environmental control
Azmacort, 101
Azobisformamide, 168

B

Bacterial infection, as asthma trigger,
    40, 49
Bahia grass pollen, 24–25
Baker's asthma, 172
Beclamethasone, 101, 129
Beclovent, 101
Belly breathing, 183, 226
Bermuda grass pollen, 24–25
Berylliosis, 175
Betamethasone, 94
Beta stimulators, 76, 225
    administration of, 104–105
    for asthma emergency, 140
    breast feeding and, 88, 131
    effect on surgery and anesthesia,
        120
    effects on mother and fetus, 129
    exercise-induced asthma and, 159
    as first-line medication, 103
    habit-forming potential, 88
    inhaled, 84, 104
    injectable, 86
    method of action, 82–83
    oral, 85, 104
    overuse of nebulized type, status
        asthmaticus development and,
        135–136
    prevention of postoperative
        complications, 123
    side effects, 87
    solutions for machine-driven

nebulization, 83
    what doctor should know before
        prescribing, 87
Beverages
    effects on beta stimulators, 88
    effects on cromolyn, 89
    effects on steroids, 100
    effects on theophylline, 80
Bilateral carotid body resection, 117
Biofeedback, 185, 225
Birch pollen, 23
Bitolterol, 84
Black lung disease, 175
Blocking antibody, 115
Blood gases, arterial, 138–139
Blood glucose, steroids and, 93
Body rhythms, effect on skin testing,
    64
Breast feeding, 46
    asthma medications and, 131–132
    beta stimulator usage and, 88
    cromolyn usage during, 89
    effect on infant's potential to
        develop asthma, 132
    steroid usage during, 100
Breathing, 195
    problems, considerations for first
        visit to allergist, 59
Breathing aids
    adaptors for hand-held inhalers,
        211–212
    hand-held inhalers, 211
    spinhalers, 212
Breathing-control exercises, 117
Breathing-muscle training exercises,
    117–118
Breath sounds, indications for
    hospitalization, 137
Brethaire, 84
Brethine, 85
Bricanyl, 85
Bromelain, 170
Brompheniramine, 129
Bronchial provocation test, 67, 174,
    225

Bronchial tubes, 191–192, 225
  overreactivity of, 44
Bronchioles, 192
Bronchiolitis, 51–52
Bronchitis, 51–52, 225
  differences from asthma and
      emphysema, 72–73
  differential diagnosis, 68–70
      by doctor, 70–71
Bronchodilators, 71, 76, 225
  beta stimulators. *See* Beta
      stimulators
  exercise-induced asthma and, 159
  reflux esophagitis during
      pregnancy and, 127
  theophylline. *See* Theophylline
Bronchospasm, 15, 225
  prevention of, 105
  self-help techniques, 160
Bronkaid, 84
Bronkometer, 84
Bronkosol, 83
Bruising of skin, from steroids, 96
Budesonide, 101
Buffalo hump, 93
Burning bush, 25
Burweed, 25
Byssinosis, 173–174

C

Caddis flies, 31–32
Caffeine, effect on theophylline, 80
CAMP, 77
Canada, locations for allergy causing
      pollens, 196–206
Cannabis pollen, 25
Carbohydrates, effect on
      theophylline, 80
Carbon dioxide, 225
  blood levels of, 139–140
Cardiac arrhythmias, 141

Cardiovascular complications, of
      steroids, 97
Carmine, 168
Castor-bean oil production, asthma
      from, 173
Categorization of asthma, 18
  medication and, 106
Cataracts, from steroids, 92–93
CBC, 138
Celestone, 94
Chemical fumigants, 111–112
Chemical mediators, 20
Chest
  deformity, from childhood asthma,
      49, 50
  movements, indications for
      hospitalization, 137
  physiotherapy, 117
  signs of asthma, 63
  X-ray, 66, 138
Chest-stress breathing, 183
Childhood asthma
  absenteeism and, 147–148
  day or resident camps for,
      213–218
  development and course of, 45–47
  effect on growth and development,
      49
  effects on intellectual development,
      54–55
  emotional effects of, 53–54
  facts and statistics, 43–44
  infection and, 49
  intrinsic, 37
  permanency of damage, 50
  physical effects of, 53
  resources for child and family,
      55–56
  school, special problems associated
      with, 146–155
  severity and prognosis, 45–46
  special exercises for, 118
  symptoms of, 50–52
  triggers for, 47–49
  uncontrolled, 50

use of oral beta stimulators, 104
vs. adult asthma, 44–45
Chloramine-t, 168
Chlorpheniramine, 129–130
Chromium, 169
Chronic asthma
long-acting theophylline
preparations for, 104
methods of taking drugs, 107
steroid dosages for, 91
Chronic obstructive pulmonary
disease (COPD), 225
Cigarette smoking, 70
Cilia, 191–192
Cimetadine, occupational asthma
from, 169
Classification of asthma, 224
severity of childhood asthma, 46
Classroom allergens, 152
Classroom behavior, by school-age
asthmatics, 150
Coal worker's pneumonconiosis, 175
Cocklebur, 25
Cockroaches, 31
Coffee beans, occupational asthma
and, 173
Cold, dry air, 41
Colds, asthma and, 39–40, 49
Colophony, 166–167
Common cold, as trigger for intrinsic
asthma, 39–40, 49
Congenital abnormalities, asthma
drugs associated with, 129–130
Conifers, 23
Control of asthma
environmental, 108–109
immunotherapy. See
Immunotherapy
indicators signifying asthma
getting out of control,
136–137
medications for, 102–108
self-help techniques, 117–118
Cotton dust, 173–174
Cottonwood pollen, 23

Cromolyn, 76, 88, 103, 225
administration of, 105
breast feeding and, 131
dosage of, 88–89
effects on mother and fetus, 129
habit-forming potential, 89
preparations, drugs commonly
used in, 89–90
before prescribing, what doctor
should know, 89
side effects of, 89
usage during pregnancy, 89
Croup, 51
Cushingoid state, 93
Cyanosis, 137, 225
Cyclic adenosine 3'5'
monophosphate, 77
Cyclopropane, 122
Cystic fibrosis, 52

D

Danders, animal, 31
environmental control measures,
112
Day camps for children with asthma,
213–215
Death, 14, 141–143
factors associated with increased
rate, 142–143
Decadron, 94
Decongestants, effects on mother
and fetus, 129–130
Dehumidifiers, suppliers, 221
Deltasone, 94
Dennie's line, 62
Dental surgery, asthma and, 123–124
Depression, childhood asthma and,
54
Dermagraphic skin, skin testing and,
65
De-stressors, 186–187

Development and growth of
    children, asthma and, 49
Dexamethasone, 94
Dexasone, 94
Diagnosis
    laboratory tests for, 63–67
    of occupational asthma, 174–175
    preparation for visit to allergist,
        58–59
Diaphragm, 183, 195, 225–226
Diaphragmatic breathing, 160, 226
Diazepam (Valium), 122
Diazonium salts, occupational
    asthma from, 168
Diet, at school, 152–153
Diphenhydramine, 129
Diphenylmethane diisocyanate
    (MDI), 165–166
Doctor
    allergist. *See* Allergist
    differentiation between asthma,
        bronchitis, and emphysema,
        70–71
    before prescribing beta
        stimulators, 87
    presurgical considerations for
        asthmatics and, 120
    role in school and parent working
        relationship, 154
    what your doctor should know
        before prescribing
        theophylline, 79–80
Drowsiness, from asthma
    medications, 149–150
Drugs, 37, 102–108. *See*
    Medications; *specific drugs*;
    specific medications
    anesthetic-inducing agents, 122
    for asthma, effects on mother and
        fetus, 128–130
    basic categories of, 76–77
    causing occupational asthma,
        169
    effects during breast feeding,
        131–132

effects on mother and fetus,
    128–130
effects on skin testing, 64
effects on surgery and anesthesia,
    120
first-line, 103
methods for taking, 106–107
muscle-relaxing agents, 122
noncompliance, 142
out of control, 136
postoperative, 122–123
preoperative, 122
second-line, 103
side effects, for school-age
    children, 149–150
taking at school, 149
third-line, 103
triggering extrinsic asthma, 33–34
undermedication, status
    asthmaticus development and,
    135
when to take, 77
Dust, 30–31
    consideration as trigger, 61
    from cotton, flax, or hemp,
        173–174
    environmental control measures,
        110–111
    grain, 172–173
    plant, 172–173
    wood, 171–172
Dust mites, 30–31, 110, 226
Dyes, occupational asthma from, 168

E

Ear infections, 49
Ears, signs of asthma, 63
Economic cost of asthma, 14
Eczema, 224, 226
Educational programs, 55–56
Electrolytes, 138
    steroids and, 95

Electrostatic precipitators, 110–111, 226
  suppliers, 220
Emergency situations
  in school, 152
  status asthmaticus. *See* Status asthmaticus
Emotional problems, 142
  in childhood asthma, 53–54
Emphysema, 50, 66, 226
  differences from asthma and bronchitis, 72–73
  differential diagnosis, 68–70
  by doctor, 70–71
Enflurane, 122
Environmental control, 226
  allergens suitable for, 110–113
  amount you should undertake, 109–110
  geographic relocation, 114
  methods, 37, 108–109
  of nonallergenic irritants, 113–114
  during pregnancy, 130
Environmental history, 61
Environmental factors, as triggers for intrinsic asthma, 40–42
Enzymes, causing occupational asthma, 169–170
Eosinophil, 226
Eosinophil count, 66, 72
Eosinophilia, 36–37
Ephedrine, 82, 85
  effects on mother and fetus, 129
Epidural block, 121
Epiglottis, acute, 52
Epinephrine
  congenital abnormalities and, 87
  effects on mother and fetus, 129
  inhaled, 84
Erythromycin, 130
Estrogen, 90
Ether, 122
Ethylene, 122
Ethylenediamine, 168
Eustachian tubes, 226

Evergreens, 23
Exercise-induced asthma, 156–157, 226
  causes of, 157
  childhood, 47
  description of, 156–157
  diagnosis, 158–159
  factors increasing chances of, 158
  intrinsic, 40
  recognition clues, 158
  treatment and control of, 159–161
Exercises
  breathing-control, 117
  breathing-muscle training, 117–118
  for children, 118
Exercise test, 158–159
Expiration, 190
Extrinsic asthma, 18, 226
  causes of, 19
  characteristics of, 38
  childhood, triggers in, 48
  differences with intrinsic asthma, 36–38
  immune system and, 20
  similarities with intrinsic asthma, 35–36
  triggers for, 21–34
Eyes
  side effects from steroids, 92–93
  signs of asthma, 62

F

Failure to treat, status asthmaticus development and, 135
Family, resources for childhood asthma, 55–56
Family history, 17–18, 60–61
  intrinsic asthma and, 36
Fat distribution, steroids and, 93, 95
FD&C Yellow #5, 37, 230
Fear, childhood asthma and, 54

Feathers, 32
  environmental control measures,
    113
Fentanyl (Sublimaze), 122
Fetus, effects of asthma on, 128
FEV_1, 71
Fever, 49
Field moulds, 28–29
Flaviastase, 170
Flax dust, 173–174
Flu, as asthma trigger, 39–40, 49
Fluid therapy, 140
Flunisolide, 101
Flu vaccines, 107
Food intolerance, 32
Foods
  effects on beta stimulators, 88
  effects on cromolyn, 89
  effects on steroids, 100
  effects on theophylline, 80
  families of, 208–210
  triggering asthma, 32–33
    in children, 47–49
Forced expiratory volume in one
    second (FEV_1), 67, 226
Forced vital capacity (FVC), 67, 226
Formaldehyde, 111–112
  occupational asthma from,
    167–168
Freon, 168
Fumes, inhaled metal salt, 169
Fumigation of room, 111–112
Fungi, causing occupational asthma,
    171

G

Gas exchange, 190
  description of process, 193–195
Gastrointestinal side effects, from
    steroids, 93
General allergy products
    information, 221

General anesthesia, 121
  adverse effect on asthma, 121–122
General health care, poor, 142
Geographic relocation, as
    environmental control, 114
Grain, causing occupational asthma,
    172–173
Grass pollens, locations in United
    States and Canada, 196–206
Growth
  childhood asthma and, 49, 53
  suppression, steroids and, 95–96

H

Halothane, 122
Hand-held inhalers, 211
  adaptors for, 104, 211–212
Hay fever, 37
Hearing loss, childhood asthma and,
    152
Heartbeat, 50
Heartburn, during pregnancy, 127
Height suppression, 49
Hemp dust, 173–174
HEPA filters, 111, 226–227
  suppliers, 219–220
Heredity, childhood asthma and, 45
Hexadroal, 94
Hexahydrophthalic anhydride, 166
Hexamethaline diisocyanate (HDI),
    165–166
Hexamethylenetetramine, 168
Hickory pollen, 23
High efficiency particulate air filter
    (HEPA), 111, 226–227
Himic anhydride, 166
Hirsutism, from steroids, 96
Histamine, 20
Hobby-related triggers, 61
Hospitalization
  decision, 137–138

typical experiences after admission, 138–141
House dust, 30–31
Huff and Puff Family Asthma Program, 55–56
Humidity, 41
Hydration, 140
Hydrocortisone, 94
Hydroxyzine, 129
Hypersensitive pneumonitis, 175
Hyperventilation, 117, 179, 227
  control in exercise-induced asthma, 160
  of pregnancy, 127, 128
  relationship to stress and asthma, 180–181, 181–182
  control of, 182–187
  signs and symptoms of, 181

I

IgE antibody, 19, 20, 227
  measurement by RAST test, 65
  pregnancy and, 127
  test for, 66
Immune system, 227
  extrinsic asthma and, 20
Immunoglobulins, 227
Immunoglobulin test, 66
Immunology, 227
  changes during pregnancy, 127
Immunotherapy, 44, 227
  adverse reactions, 115–116
  breast feeding and, 131–132
  controversial techniques, 116–117
  efficacy of, 114–115
  how allergy shots work, 115
  during pregnancy, 130
  success of, 116
Impaired wound healing, from steroids, 96
Incentive spirometer, 123

Industrial chemicals, causing occupational asthma, 165–168
Industrial smog, 41–42
Infant. *See also* Childhood asthma
  inheritance of asthma and, 131
  precautions to decrease incidence or delay of allergy development, 132
Infections
  respiratory, status asthmaticus development and, 135
  steroids and, 97–98
  as trigger for intrinsic asthma, 39–40
Inferiority, childhood asthma and, 54
Inhal-Aid, 104
Inhalers, hand-held, 211
  adaptors for, 211–212
Inheritance of asthma, 131
Insect particles, 31–32
Insect-pollinated plants, 22
Insects, causing occupational asthma, 170–171
Inspiration, 190
Inspirease, 104
Intrinsic asthma
  age of onset, 35
  cause of, 35
Insulin, 100
Intal. *See* Cromolyn
Intellectual development, childhood asthma and, 54–55
Intermittent occurrence of asthma, methods of taking drugs for, 106–107
Intermittent positive pressure breathing machines (IPPB), 212
Intradermal skin test, 227
Intrinsic asthma, 18, 227
  characteristics of, 38
  childhood, 45
    triggers in, 48
  differences with extrinsic asthma, 36–38

similarities with extrinsic asthma, 35–36
triggers for, 38–42
Iodides, usage during pregnancy, 130
IPPB machines, 212
Ipratropium bromide (Atrovent), 108
Irritability, from asthma medications, 149–150
Irritating substances, triggers for intrinsic asthma, 39
Isocyanates, 165–166
Isoetharine, 84
   effects on mother and fetus, 129
Isoflurane, 122
Isoproterenol (isoprenaline), 84
   effects on mother and fetus, 129
Isuprel, 83

J

Johnson grass pollen, 24–25
Jute allergen, 32, 113

K

Kerosene heaters, 114
Ketamine (Ketalar), 122
Kochia, 25

L

Laboratory tests. *See also specific laboratory tests*
   diagnostic, 63–67
   in differential diagnosis, 71
   postadmission, 138
Lambs' quarter, 25
Laryngotracheobronchitis, 51
Larynx, 191

Leukocytotoxic testing, 65
Liquid Pred syrup, 94
Local anesthesia, 121
Lung diseases, differential diagnosis, 68–70
Lungs, 191–192

M

Maple pollen, 23
Marijuana, 25
Mast cells, 20, 227
Mattress covers, 110, 221
Maxatose, 170
"Meat-wrappers" asthma, 166
Mediators, 20, 227
Medical history, 60–62
Medications. *See* Drugs; *specific medications*
Medicines, considerations for first visit to allergist, 59
Medihaler-Epi, 84
Medihaler-Iso, 84
Meditation, 185–186, 227–228
Medrol, 94
Menstrual irregularities, steroids and, 95
Mental function, indication for hospitalization, 137
Meperidine (Demerol), 122
Metabolic acidosis, status asthmaticus and, 136
Metabolic side effects, from steroids, 93, 95–96
Metacholine pulmonary function test, 228
Metal salts, 168–169
Metaprel, 84, 85
Metaproterenol (orciprenaline), 84, 85
   effects on mother and fetus, 129
Methacholine challenge test, 159
Methohexital (Brevitol), 122

Methyl dopa, occupational asthma from, 169
Methylprednisolone, 94
  intravenous, 140
  troleandomycin and, 106
Midazolam (Versed), 122
Mild asthma, 224
Mites, dust, 30–31
Moderate asthma, 224
  steroid dosages for, 91
"Monday morning fever", 173
Monoethanolamine, 168
Moon face, 93
Morbidity, 228
Morphine, 122
Mortality, 14, 228
Mortality rate, 141–143
Motorized nebulizers, 104, 212
Mould, 28–29, 228
  consideration as trigger, 61
  indoor, environmental control of, 111–112
  outdoor, environmental control measures, 112
  as trigger for asthma, 207
Mountain cedar, 23
Mouth, signs of asthma, 63
Mucous secretions, inability to clear by coughing, 136
Mucus, 191
Muscle relaxation, progressive, 184–185
Muscle-relaxing agents, 122
Musculoskeletal side effects, from steroids, 96–97
Myopathy, 97

N

Naphthylene diisocyanate (NDI), 165–166
Nasal congestion, 37, 72
Nasal inflammation, during

pregnancy, 127–128
Nasal polyps, 37, 228
Nasal smear, 66
Nebulization of beta stimulators, 140
Nebulizers, 228
  motorized, 104, 212
Nerve block, 121
Nervous system side effects, from steroids, 92
Nickel, 169
Nitrogen dioxide, 42
Nonalcoholic beverages
  effects on beta stimulators, 88
  effects on cromolyn, 89
  effects on theophylline, 80
Nonallergenic irritants, environmental control of, 113–114
Nonallergic asthma. See Intrinsic asthma
Nonallergic reactions, from occupational asthma, 165
Nonmedical treatment of asthma, 142
Nonsteroidal anti-inflammatory drugs, 37, 228
  steroids and, 99
Nose, 191
  signs of asthma, 62–63
Nursing mothers, use of theophylline, 80

O

Oak pollen, 23
Occupational asthma, 162–163
  causative agents, 61, 165–174
  developmental factors, 163–164
  diagnosis of, 174–175
  importance of classification, 164
  prevention, 176
  reactions from, 164–165
  treatment, 175–176

Occupations, associated with
  isocyanate agents, 166
Occupational asthma, 228
Odors, triggering intrinsic asthma,
  39, 113
Orciprenaline (metaproterenol), 84,
  85, 129
Osteoporosis, 96–97
Over-the-counter drugs, 37
Oxygen, 190
Oxygen blood levels, 139
Oxygen therapy, 141
Ozone, 42

P

Pancreatic enzymes, 170
Papain, 170
Paraformaldehyde, 111–112
Paraphenylenediamine, 168
Parasympathetic nervous system, 228
Parent, guidelines for working with
  school, 153–155
Peak flowmeter, 67, 159
Pediapred, 94
Peer-group pressure, of school-age
  asthmatics, 148–149
Penicillin
  allergy to, 33–34
  usage during pregnancy, 130
Penicillin-class drugs, occupational
  asthma from, 169
Penicillium, 28, 34
Pepsin, 170
Personality changes, from steroids,
  92
Persulfates, 168
pH, blood, 139–140
Phenylephrine, 129
Phenylglycine acid chloride,
  occupational asthma from, 169
Phenylpropanolamine, 129
Photochemical smog, 42

Phthalic anhydride, 166
Physical education class,
  participation in, 150–151
Physical effects, of childhood asthma,
  53
Physical examination, 62–63
Physical signs, in differential
  diagnosis, 71
Physician. See Doctor
Pigweed, 25
Pillow covers, 113, 221
Piperazine, occupational asthma
  from, 169
Plantain, 25
Plant dust, causing occupational
  asthma, 172–173
Plant fibres, 32
Plants
  insect-pollinated, 22
  wind-pollinated, 22
Platinum salts, 168–169
Plicatic acid, 171
Pneumoconiosis, coal worker's, 175
Pneumomediastinum, 138, 141, 229
Pneumonia, 49, 138, 229
Pneumothorax, 138, 141, 229
Pollen, 229
  environmental control measures,
    112–113
  grass, 24–25
  locations in United States and
    Canada, 196–206
  triggering extrinsic asthma, 22–28
  weed, 25, 28
Pollen count, 22, 229
Pollination, 229
Poplar pollen, 23
Postoperative complications,
  prevention, 123
Postoperative medications, 122–123
Posture, childhood asthma and, 53
Prednisolone, 94
Prednisone, 90, 229
  duration and potency, 94
  prolonged usage, 105–106

stopping of drug, 106
time required to work, 91–92
Pregnancy
  asthma and, 125–126
  beta stimulator usage during,
    87–88
  chances of infant getting asthma,
    131
  cromolyn usage during, 89
  effects of asthma on mother and
    fetus, 128
  effects on asthma, 127–128
  management of asthma during,
    130–131
  normal changes during, effect on
    asthma, 126–127
  steroid usage during, 100
  theophylline usage during, 80
Prelone syrup, 94
Preoperative drugs, 122
Prevention, occupational asthma, 176
Primatine, 84
Progestins, 90
Prognosis, 70
Progressive muscle relaxation, 160,
  184–185, 229
Protein, effect on theophylline, 80
Proventil, 83, 84, 85
Pseudephedrine (Sudafed), 128–130
Psychosomatic, 229
Psyllium, occupational asthma from,
  169
Pulmonary function tests, 67, 138,
  229
  for differential diagnosis, 71
Pyrethrum, 32, 113

Q

Questions about your condition, 59

R

Radioallergosorbent test (RAST),
  65, 229

Ragweed, 25, 113
Rain, 41
RAST test, 65, 229
Recess, childhood asthmatics and,
  151–152
Recognition of asthma, by school,
  147
Reflex bronchospasm, 41, 229
Reflux esophagitis, during pregnancy,
  127
Relaxation techniques, for exercise-
  induced asthma, 160
Relaxed breathing (diaphragmatic
  breathing), 183–184, 226
Remissions, 37
Resentment, childhood asthma and,
  54
Resident camps for children with
  asthma, 215–218
Respiration, 190
Respiratory system
  basic function of, 190–191
  components of, 191–193
  disorders caused by exposure in
    workplace, 175
  infections, status asthmaticus
    development and, 135
  postoperative complications, 123
  viral infection, as trigger for
    childhood asthma, 47
Rhinitis, during pregnancy, 127–128
Rinkel method, 65–66, 117
Roxane, 94
Russian thistle, 25

S

Sage, 25
Salbutamol (albuterol), 84, 85
  effects on mother and fetus, 129
Salicylate, 37
School
  common problems faced by
    asthmatics, 147–153

guidelines for parent working
 with, 153–155
recognition of asthma existence in
 child, 147
understanding and action, 147
Scratch test, 63–64, 229
Seasonal variation, 19
Seizures, 143
Self-help techniques
 for control of asthma, 117–118
 for exercise-induced asthma, 160
Sensitizers, 162, 163
Severe asthma, 224
 steroid dosages for, 91
Severity
 of asthma attacks, 16–17
  blood-gas measurements and,
   139
  during pregnancy, 126
 of byssinosis, 174
 classifications for childhood
  asthma, 46
 of status asthmaticus, 133–135,
  143
 of symptoms at night, 15
Shock, 141
Signs. See Symptoms
Signs or symptoms, physical
 examination for, 62–63
Silicosis, 175
Sinusitis, 37, 49, 66, 229
Sinus X-ray, 66–67
Skin
 problems from steroids, 96
 signs of asthma, 63
Skin tests, 36, 63–64, 229
 factors affecting, 64–65
Smog, 41–42
Smoking, 68, 72, 113. See also
 Tobacco
 history of, in differential diagnosis,
  70–71
Social and emotional history, 61–62
Social problems, 142
Somatopsychic, 230

Spinhalers, 212
Spiramycin, occupational asthma
 from, 169
Sports, exercise-induced asthma. See
 Exercise-induced asthma
Sprints, warm-up for exercise-
 induced asthma, 159–160
Sputum smear, 66
Statistics on asthma, 14
 during childhood, 43–44
 status asthmaticus, 134–135
Status asthmaticus, 50, 230
 dangerous complications of, 141
 factors associated with
  development of, 135–136
 severity, 143
 severity and danger of, 133–135
 statistics, 134–135
Steroids, 76, 90–91, 223, 230
 activity in body, 91
 breast feeding and, 131
 dosages, 91
 effect on surgery and anesthesia,
  120–121
 effects on intake of food,
  beverages, and tobacco, 100
 effects on growth and development
  of children, 49
 effects on mother and fetus, 129
 habit-forming potential, 100
 how long does it take to work,
  91–92
 inadequate doses, 142
 inadequate usage of, status
  asthmaticus development and,
  135
 inhaled, 100–101, 103
 oral, 103, 105–106
 prescribing, what your doctor
  should know, 99
 side effects, 92–93, 95–99
  most common, 98–99
  treatment, 99
 stopping of, side effects related to,
  98

systemic, 140
types of, 90–91
Storage moulds, 28
Stress, 230
  asthma, hyperventilation and,
    177–178, 181–182
  control of, 182–187
  causes of, 179–180
  definition of, 178–179
  internal effects of, 179
  signs and symptoms of, 180
  status asthmaticus and, 136
  as trigger for intrinsic asthma, 40
Stress, asthma and, 53
Stress breathing, 230
Stressors, 178–179, 230
Striae, from steroids, 96
Subcutaneous provocation testing,
  65
Subcutaneous testing, 117
Sublingual provocation testing, 65,
  117
Sudafed (pseudephedrine), 128
Sulfites, 33, 230
Sulfur dioxide, 42, 114
Suppliers
  dehumidifiers, 221
  of electrostatic precipitators, 220
  of HEPA filters, 219–220
  mattress and pillow enclosures,
    221
Suptum exam, 138
Surgery
  dental, 123–124
  doctor, presurgical considerations,
    120
  postoperative respiratory
    complications, 123
  presurgical considerations,
    119–120
Sweat chloride test, 66, 230
Sweating, from steroids, 96
Sycamore pollen, 23
Sympathetic nervous system,
  230

Sympathomimetic bronchodilators,
  83
Symptoms, 15
  inability to control, 136
  of intrinsic asthma, 35, 36
  of occupational asthma, 162–163
  pattern of, 72
  patterns of, in differential
    diagnosis, 71
  recognition in childhood asthma,
    50–52
  severity at night, 15

T

Tartrazine, 37, 230
Terbutaline, 84, 85
  effects on mother and fetus, 129
Testosterone, 90
Tetrachloraphthalic anhydride
  (TCPA), 166
Tetracycline, 130
  occupational asthma from, 169
Tetrazene, 168
Theophylline, 76, 230
  absorption of, 78–79
  activity of, 77
  breast feeding and, 131
  dosage, 77–78
  effect on surgery and anesthesia,
    120
  effects on mother and fetus, 129
  exercise-induced asthma and, 159
  forms of, 78
  habit-forming potential, 80
  intravenous, 140
  loading dose, 140
  maximum effect of, 78–79
  preparations, drugs used in, 81–82
  serum level, 138
  side effects, 79
  use as first-line medication, 103
  use by nursing mothers, 80

use during pregnancy, 80
what your doctor should know
before prescribing, 79–80
when to take, 103–104
Thinning of skin, from steroids, 96
Thiopenthal (Pentothal), 122
Tobacco. *See also* Smoking
effects on beta stimulators, 88
effects on cromolyn, 89
effects on theophylline, 80
steroids and, 100
as trigger for intrinsic asthma, 39
Toluene diisocyanate (TDI), 165–166
Tonsils, 63
Tornalate, 84
Toxicity
of beta stimulators, 87
of theophylline, 79
Trachea, 191
Transilluminator, 63
Treatment. *See also* Control of asthma
of exercise-induced asthma,
159–161
goals for, 102
in hospital, 138–140
immunotherapy. *See*
Immunotherapy
medications for control of asthma,
102–108
of occupational asthma, 175–176
during pregnancy, 130–131
self-help techniques, 117–118
Tree pollens, 22–23
locations in United States and
Canada, 196–206
Triamcinolone, 94, 101
Triggers, 17, 230. *See also specific*
triggers
in childhood asthma, 47–49
elimination. *See* Environmental
control
for extrinsic asthma, 21–34
for intrinsic asthma, 38–42
Trimellitic anhydride, 166
Tripelennamine, 130

Troleandomycin, 130
methylprednisolone and, 106
Trypsin, 170
Tumbleweed, 25

U

Uncontrolled asthma attacks, during
pregnancy, 126
Undermedication, status asthmaticus
development and, 135
United States
day camps for children with
asthma, 213–215
locations for allergy-causing
pollens, 196–206
resident camps for children with
asthma, 215–218

V

Valium (diazepam), 122
Vanadium, 169
Vanceril, 101
Vasomotor rhinitis, 230
of pregnancy, 127–128
Vegetable gum dust asthmas, 173
Ventolin, 83, 84, 85
Versed (midazolam), 122
Viral infection, as asthma trigger,
39–40, 47, 49
Visualization, 230
as de-stressor, 187
in progressive muscle relaxation,
184–185
of relaxed breathing, 184
Vital capacity, 71
Vital signs, indicating need for
hospitalization, 137

W

Walnut pollen, 23

Warm-up sprints, exercise-induced asthma and, 159–160
Water changes, steroids and, 95
Weather, as trigger for intrinsic asthma, 40–41
Weed pollens, 25, 28
  locations in United States and Canada, 196–206
Weight gain, steroids and, 93
Western red cedar dust, 171
Western water hemp, 25
Wheeze, 137, 230
Willow pollen, 23
Wind, 41
Windpipes, 191–192
Wind-pollinated plants, 22
  trees, 23

Wood dust, causing occupational asthma, 171–172
Wool, 113
Workplace
  development of asthma in. *See* Occupational asthma
  lung conditions associated with, 175

X

X-rays
  chest, 66
  in differential diagnosis, 71
  sinus, 66–67